Who says a good diet has to be dull?

- Cornish Game Hens Dijonnaise, raspberries in champagne, Lamb Provençal, caviar omelettes . . . *The Snowbird Diet* offers you delightful gourmet dishes that are easy to prepare.

- A fitness program that is not only healthful, but fun . . . *The Snowbird Diet* teaches you how to experience exercise as play.

- The expertise of an entire staff of health specialists from Dr. Robertson's center . . . *The Snowbird Diet* gives you the advice and guidance of a psychologist, dietician, nutritionist, and exercise physiologist. You'll learn how to unlock the secrets of your metabolism and motivate yourself through imagery and progress records.

- An emergency diet plan that lets you travel, eat out, go to parties, entertain at home . . . *The Snowbird Diet* lets you enjoy your lifestyle.

- A maintenance plan that lets you enjoy special treats, plan for "hungry" times, and enjoy a normal social life . . . *The Snowbird Diet* is realistic, flexible, personalized, positive—and can lead to a lifetime of low weight!

"Diet has always been a four-letter word, but now it's synonymous with haute cuisine."
—Dorothy Goebel, Living Editor, *Phoenix Gazette*

The recipes shown on the cover are Veal Chops with Salsa of Peppers (page 102), Sonora Salad (page 122) and Strawberries with Mint (page 122).

THE
SNOWBIRD
DIET

12 Days to a Slender Future—
And a Lifetime of Gourmet Dining

Donald S. Robertson, M.D., M.Sc.
and Carol P. Robertson

WARNER BOOKS

A Warner Communications Company

Ⓦ A Warner Communications Company

Printed in the United States of America
First Printing: February 1986
10 9 8 7 6 5 4 3 2 1

Library of Congress Cataloging in Publication Data

Robertson, Donald S.
  The snowbird diet.

  Bibliography: p. 280
  Includes index.
  1. Reducing diets—Recipes.   2. Reducing exercises.
3. Reducing—Psychological aspects.   I. Robertson, Carol P.
II. Title.
RM222.2.R57   1986   613.2'5   84-40436
ISBN 0-446-38283-3 (U.S.A.) (pbk.)
ISBN 0-446-38284-1 (Canada) (pbk.)

Book design: H. Roberts Design

To Cathy, who has helped change the lives of so many

ACKNOWLEDGMENTS

We wish most especially to thank George L. Blackburn, M.D., Ph.D., and Peter G. Lindner, M.D. Their expertise, encouragement, research data, and clinical experience in the field of nutrition and weight control not only made this mid-life career change possible but an ongoing reality. For this and for their friendship and stimulation we remain everlastingly grateful.

Heartfelt thanks to Mary Ruth Wilde, whose superb hard work was surpassed only by her extraordinary results.

We are particularly indebted to Sue Olson; Jeanne Patterson; Karen Winden; Paula Wolfert; Charlotte Kuentz; and Cheryl Bronkesh. We wish to thank Kathleen and Julie Martin for their meticulous standization of the recipes in this book. Our thanks also to Rosalee Barker; La Donne Batty; Barbara Bonoff; Nancy Chaboun; Joan Conlon; Melinda Cory; Freida's Finest Produce Specialties, Inc.; Dorothy Goebel; Dalma Heyn; Ken Horn; Sandy Koons; Carol Lynn Kroger; Carol Ladner; Jill Landis; Ginny Mahlios; Jane Matyas; Zibby Miles; Rita Mulholland; Janet Nazzaro; Cindy Pratt; Midge Schildkraut; The Silver Palate; Robin Spotleson; Carol Steele; Mary Toscus; Larry Wilde; and Richard Wohl. Our special thanks to our tireless agent, Jane Jordan Browne, and her able assistant, Greg Getschman, for their endless patience, and last but certainly not least, every author's dream, the perfect editor, Patti Breitman.

CONTENTS

Part III

Essentials for Success

Part IV

The Keys to a Slender Lifetime
               or
Nothing Tastes as Good as This Feels

INTRODUCTION

As medical director of the Southwest Bariatric Nutrition Center for the past seven years, and an internist specializing in gastroenterology for twenty-five years, I've had a front-row seat for all kinds of food-related maladies.

My work in bariatric medicine (the treatment of adult obesity) here in Scottsdale lets me see the effects of fad dieting firsthand.

By the time I treat them, most of my patients have been on dozens of fad diets. Here are the results: they are overweight, undernourished, and out of shape. Their bodies are so badly out of tune they *can't* burn off fat.

So how do I treat the ills of unhealthful, unenlightened living?

Well, that brings us to the Snowbird Diet.

But before I tell you what the Snowbird Diet **is**, let me tell you what it is **not**.

It is **not** another fad diet.

It is **not** a two-week blitz that will eventually lead to more fat and frustration.

It is **not** a nutritionally impoverished gimmick that leads you to think you've lost *fat*, when actually you've lost critical *body fluids* and lean *muscle tissue*.

It is **not** an overnight wonder that promises to incinerate pounds as if by magic. (When a diet sounds too good to be true, it usually is.)

It is **not a media** maneuver to give you sensational but artificial weight loss with no chance whatsoever to keep it off.

Studies show that 95 percent of people who go on fad diets fail miserably. Of the 5 percent who manage to lose 40 pounds, less than 1 percent are able to keep it off even up to one year. That's a .005 percent success rate.

The Snowbird Diet is **not** a fad diet.

Fad diets don't work.

The Snowbird Diet is a new, lifetime weight-management plan. **It works!**

Over 80 percent of the patients who remain in the program at the Southwest Bariatric Nutrition Center, where the Snowbird Diet was developed, lose 40 pounds or more. And over 30 percent have kept the weight off.* That's about 600 times better than the national average.

Now let me tell you what the Snowbird Diet **is**.

It is a plan formulated by top experts in weight management and related fields—bariatrics, nutrition, exercise physiology, psychology, and even haute cuisine, based on the famous, highly successful program at the Southwest Bariatric Nutrition Center in Scottsdale, Arizona.

It is a *complete* medical weight-loss program that integrates fat loss with fitness, preventive medicine, and life extension.

It is a safe, scientific, and highly motivating plan that offers real hope for permanent weight management.

It is a plan that treats overweight for what it really is—or could be: a serious medical disease.

This is the first time that this program has been made available to the general public.

The Snowbird Diet is for active, high-powered people who want to travel, entertain, dine out, and enjoy a good life, yet keep trim and fit.

The Snowbird Diet is an intelligent approach to weight reduction.

It is simple, yet sophisticated, well respected, medically sound, nutritionally balanced, thoughtful, and sensitive, and its principles have helped hundreds of people lose thousands of pounds.

I am confident it can work for you.

Read it carefully from cover to cover before you begin. All the

* Based on a three-year study. A five-year study is in progress.

components of the Snowbird Diet work in concert with one another to achieve lasting weight reduction. No one component stands alone.

Use it as prescribed. Make it part of your life. Act as if your life depended on it. It does.

The Snowbird Diet can prove to you once and for all that you can live a slender life. You can operate at your maximum potential. You can feel like a million. And best of all, once you learn its secrets, you will never have to be fat again.

Congratulations,

Donald S. Robertson

Donald S. Robertson, M.D., M.Sc.
Medical Director
Southwest Bariatric Nutrition Center
Scottsdale, Arizona

PART I

The Snowbird Diet:
12 Days to a
Slender Lifetime

1

A Private Clinic Shares Its Secrets

Snowbird is a term usually used to describe flocks of frostbitten, sun-starved northerners who fly south each winter looking for rejuvenation of body and spirit.

Snowbirds of a special sort have been flocking to the Southwest Bariatric Nutrition Center in Scottsdale, Arizona, for the past seven years. They come from around the state, across the country, and around the world, not only to escape the chill of winter but to find relief from a more painful and perplexing problem—overweight.

When they arrive, most of them look and feel older than their years. Many suffer from a long list of ills related to overweight, including depression, hypertension, and diabetes, to name a few. But when they leave, most are trim, fit, and revitalized.

That's why *Snowbird* is the name of the diet developed at the Southwest Bariatric Nutrition Center. The name is appropriate because its principles for weight loss are uncommonly successful at revitalizing and rejuvenating both the body and the spirit.

The changes that take place when a patient loses a lot of weight are not just physical. There's a kind of emotional metamorphosis as well. Self-image can be dramatically altered. Very often a happier, more positive, more dynamic human being emerges from under the layers of fat. The dieter is "lighter" both physically and mentally.

Here is how some patients express their new outlook:

"I didn't know a diet could feel so great."

"I'm very proud of myself. For the first time, I have lost weight and kept it off."

"I'm wearing clothes I never thought I'd fit into again."

"Everyone says I look younger. And you know what? I *feel* younger."

"This program has really simplified my life. It's so automatic now I don't even have to think about it."

"It feels great to be able to buy fashionable clothes in a small size."

"All my friends keep asking me what miracle diet I've been on."

"I'm not hungry. And I have more energy than I've had in years."

"I was out with my husband and one of my friends didn't stop to say hello. She thought he was out with another woman."

"I don't need as much sleep now, and I never nap during the day."

"My family is delighted that I feel so good about myself."

HOW THE SNOWBIRD WAS HATCHED

The Southwest Bariatric Nutrition Center came about like so many things in life—through a series of unplanned events.

In 1977 my 17-year-old stepdaughter, Cathy, was suffering from a severe weight problem. After a kidney transplant at age 9 she had steadily gained weight. By the time she was 17, it had become a source of tremendous frustration, upset, and physical disability.

She tried the usual assortment of diets, but the results were always the same—she'd lose a little and gain it back.

My wife, Carol, and I took Cathy to one expert after another. Psychiatrists, medical doctors, dieticians—but none offered any long-term help.

Looking back on it, the most disheartening moment came in the office of a top endocrinologist. He said, "I don't think your daughter *can* lose much weight. She'll probably be fighting this the rest of her life."

Cathy simply would not give up. She wanted to be thin more than anything. And we were bound to help her achieve her goal.

My search led to a revolutionary new weight-loss program in Boston. It was run by George Blackburn, M.D., Ph.D., and associate professor of surgery at Harvard Medical School.

With the facilities and personnel of Harvard and M.I.T. behind him, Dr. Blackburn had an impressive volume of research and data to back up his incredibly successful program.

Here was an enormously respected physician pioneering in weight control—an area treated with contempt by so many doctors. Yet Dr. Blackburn was treating obesity as a serious medical problem, using the latest research, nutritional data, and equipment available.

Our lives were about to be changed drastically.

That fall, Cathy enrolled in college in Boston. She also became one of Dr. Blackburn's patients.

Imagine our jubilance when six months later she stepped off the plane a total of 37 pounds lighter! Since Cathy was only 4 feet 6 inches tall, that kind of weight loss was even more astounding.

Until this time I was a practicing internist and gastroenterologist. I became so interested in bariatric medicine (the treatment of obesity) that I knew the course of my life would be changed forever.

In 1978 I opened the Southwest Bariatric Nutrition Center in Scottsdale, Arizona. The program is based on the prototype in Boston. It offers periodic medical evaluations, weekly monitoring, education classes, self-image workshops, and, most important, a strong maintenance program.

The Town That Lost a Ton

In no time, the patient roster blossomed by word of mouth. In "The Town That Lost a Ton," an article written by Dalma Heyn in the

January 1981 issue of *McCall's* magazine, you get an idea of how the clinic expanded:

> Every Tuesday, Cheryl . . . left Bagdad, the tiny Arizona copper-mining town she lives in, by six sharp. She could cover the 130-mile drive to Scottsdale in three hours and arrive at the Southwest Bariatric Nutrition Center in time for her nine-o'clock appointment with Dr. Robertson. . . .
>
> By the end of the sixteenth week, Cheryl had lost 70 pounds.
>
> She began the program in August . . . by December, Cheryl was very slim, a fact that did not go unnoticed in Bagdad. There was no doubt that this thing Cheryl was doing, whatever it was, was working.
>
> That was enough to sell the program to Cheryl's good friend, Lenise M. . . .
>
> It worked well for Lenise. She went from 156 to 122. . . .
>
> Soon a parade of once-skeptical Bagdadians—twenty-three women and nine men—were traipsing in and out of the Southwest Bariatric Nutrition Center, gladly surrendering their bodies, a good portion of them anyway, to Dr. Robertson.

Success Stories

At the clinic, before and after files are piled high. Photographs visually illustrate how astonishing the physical changes can be. Yet, I am more fascinated by the improvement in the *quality* of the patients' lives.

Let me share some of the successes that make work at the Southwest Bariatric Nutrition Center so gratifying to me.

Stephanie M.

Stephanie was a somewhat successful stockbroker whose career and social life had stopped blossoming. Her weight had climbed to 240 pounds. She was depressed, fatigued, highly stressed, and afraid that she could no longer keep up with the demands of her job.

Having heard about the Southwest Bariatric Nutrition Center from a business associate, she came here hoping to solve her weight problem. Little did any of us know to what extent that would eventually change her life!

From the moment she started the program, her outlook was visibly improved. A more dynamic Stephanie began to emerge.

Within the first three months, with a weight loss of 50 pounds, she became the top salesperson in her firm. She went on to lose a total of 97 pounds.

Today she is not only slim and attractive, but this energetic bundle is also one of the top stockbrokers in the Southwest.

Paul R.

Paul was a high-powered, extremely successful entrepreneur who could easily run a huge corporation. Yet he could not take charge of his own life.

In fact, his weight had become so unmanageable that Paul later admitted he had been sure he would die before reaching the age of 45.

When he came to the Southwest Bariatric Nutrition Center he was 41 and weighed 330 pounds. His blood pressure, cholesterol, triglycerides, and blood-sugar levels were dangerously high. Yet, even though his cardiac risk factors were gravely elevated, Paul did not come to the clinic for health reasons.

What motivated him?

A brand-new bright red Ferrari.

His wife had given him the luxurious sports car for his birthday. It was the wrong size. Paul simply couldn't squeeze into it, and Ferrari didn't make anything larger.

He sold his dream car and checked into the clinic the following week.

One year later, a slim Paul rewarded himself with another Ferrari, and this time it fit. He had lost to goal and his cardiac risk factors were normal.

Today Paul maintains his weight with the same careful attention and enthusiasm with which he operates his business—and his sports cars.

Eliza D.

At 175 pounds, Eliza was no longer the cheerful, vigorous restaurateur she had once been. As her business had expanded, so had her figure.

When a major magazine published an article about the restaurant, Eliza was devastated. The reviews were good and the publicity was invaluable. But the photograph of her revealed just how much weight she had gained. She hadn't realized she'd changed so much.

Eliza did what lots of people do—she went on a crash diet. It didn't work. She tried another. It, too, failed. She got fatter and more frustrated.

When she finally came to the Southwest Bariatric Nutrition Center, she was taking prescriptions for depression and hypertension.

Within three weeks of starting the program, Eliza was able to stop taking the antidepressants. As her weight dropped, so did her anxiety level and her blood pressure.

Being in the food business might be considered a dangerous occupation for a person with a weight problem. Yet Eliza has managed to maintain her weight loss. She has stated that the program actually helped refine her sense of taste.

Clearly, Eliza's case illustrates that one can enjoy fine food and still be slender.

Philip W.

Philip W. was a successful builder, with a growing business, a lovely wife, and a fine home, and he was well respected in the community. There were only two pieces of the puzzle missing. Philip and his wife were unable to conceive a child, and his weight was out of control. It did not occur to him that the problems might be related.

When he came to the Southwest Bariatric Nutrition Center, he was 90 pounds overweight.

While he was in the process of losing the weight, he and his wife adopted a baby.

Shortly after he left the clinic, having lost to goal, he and his wife conceived a child.

Could losing weight have improved his fertility? It's entirely possible. Studies have shown that the testosterone levels may drop significantly in overweight males.

The Clinic's Program Goes Public

As I mentioned earlier, patients at the Southwest Bariatric Nutrition Center come from all over the United States and many other countries. Many of these patients leave families and businesses behind for weeks, even months.

Eventually they must return to their homes and careers, sometimes before they have lost to goal. So, the question arose:

What's the best way to treat patients who are not under the clinic's strict medical supervision?

The obvious solution was to create a plan that they could take with them to be used at home or away from home.

However, capturing on the printed page what we do here at the clinic proved to be a very tall order.

In essence, the idea was to adapt the techniques, methods, and principles used at the clinic for simple, effective use by anyone.

Sounds simple. But here are just a few of the considerations.

Goals of the Diet's Creators

• *To impart the same standards of excellence as those for which the clinic has become known.*

• *To be based on sound, medically proven, respected techniques.*

• *To be nutritionally safe and sound.* Gimmicks fail the patient in the long run. We did not want to risk damaging the credibility and respectability of the Southwest Bariatric Nutrition Center.

• *To be convenient.* Just because a person is overweight does not mean he or she should stop entertaining, dining out, traveling, and socializing. This plan does not set up roadblocks to living.

• *To be simple.* So many of our patients are high-powered people with active and varied lifestyles. This diet was formulated to complement a busy schedule.

• *To be exciting.* Patients have had their fill of boring, monotonous diets. Many patients are well traveled and have dined in the world's finest restaurants. For them to stay enthused about *any* diet, the food must be extraordinary.

• *To appeal to reason and intellect.* Most patients have had it with superficial diets. They are a waste of time and energy. So, instead of insisting on blind faith, the Snowbird Diet explains how the program works, why it works, and how the patient can make it work.

• *To attack fat from every angle*—just like the Southwest Bariatric Nutrition Center does. Diet is *not* the most important part. Permanent weight loss happens only with a well-rounded program.

After years of research, planning, and work, the Snowbird Diet was formulated for use by the general public.

Like its parent, the program at the Southwest Bariatric Nutrition Center, it has all the necessary ingredients for lifelong weight control.

It is safe, satisfying, sensible, sophisticated, scientific, and simple.

Why Most Diets Don't Work

You may be feeling a little scared that this program won't work for you. That fear is only natural. If you are one of the millions who have tried some of the recent popular diets, your fear of failure may be well founded.

It's worth mentioning again: statistics show that 95 percent of those who go on fad diets fail to lose weight. And of the 5 percent who lose 40 pounds, less than 1 percent are able to maintain it for up to one year. That's a .005 percent success rate.

What does this prove?

In our opinion, it suggests that *you are not failing the diet, the diet is failing you.*

Why do so many diets fail?

• *They are nutritionally deficient.* Many have been concocted by nonprofessionals or those interested in quick weight loss for a quick buck.

To bring on this sort of weight loss, entire food groups are severely restricted or eliminated.

This results in a malnourished body.

A malnourished body cannot metabolize (burn) fat at its maximum potential. Thus, when your diet is nutritionally deficient, you can't burn off fat as well as you should.

To complicate matters, unsound nutrition can induce depression, listlessness, and fatigue, which very often compel the dieter to binge.

• *They are totally unrealistic.* Who in his right mind, overweight or not, can face a lifetime of monotonous, spartan meals without wanting to cheat? Like it or not, food equals fun and love in our culture. Any diet that treats food as a crime or a punishment is doomed to fail.

• *They force you to lose weight too quickly.* The quick-weight-loss scheme appeals to so many dieters. They believe they are losing fat. In reality, what is lost is mostly critical body fluids and muscle tissue—*not* just fat.

These diets rely on food gimmicks. When the body is improperly nourished, it begins to use up muscle as well as fat. Having lost lean body tissue, the minute you resume your usual eating patterns, you frequently put back more weight, ending up with more fat and less lean body mass. As you can see, this is totally counterproductive.

• *They do not address all the issues.* Most focus on only one or two aspects of losing weight—usually diet and exercise. You may stick to the plan religiously for a few weeks, but when the chips are down, there is no maintenance plan to fall back on. Can you maintain weight loss without a good solid maintenance plan? Fat chance!

• *They are monotonous.* And monotony is a dieter's downfall. The same humdrum foods day after day. The same robotic exercises over and over. No wonder you're looking for a new diet. You're bored to tears!

• *They are too difficult.* Some dieters are so determined to lose weight that they would stand on their ears if they thought it would make them shed a pound. But in the long run, most diets make it too difficult for a person to stick with it.

Recently I treated a patient from Los Angeles. She had been on a popular fad diet in which some of the required foods were exotic, seasonal produce. In the middle of her diet, she was forced to go out of the country on a business trip.

Afraid that the necessary foods might not be available, she "smuggled" a carry-on bag full of fruit onto the plane. A week later she had nothing to show for her trouble but a bag full of fruit flies. She was off the diet and on to foods available in restaurants.

Obviously, this diet was not convenient in any but the most controlled circumstances.

• *They do not make the patient feel good.* So many dieters abandon a weight-loss plan because they feel hungry, weak, lackluster, sluggish, constipated, ravenous, deprived, flabby, and haggard. Again, this is due primarily to poor nutrition and inadequate fluid intake, but it can also be caused by a diet that fails to treat the emotional side of losing weight.

The reason most diets you've tried haven't worked is the diet's fault—not yours.

People cannot and should not be expected to cure themselves of a potentially serious medical problem without proper, medically based, nutritionally sound treatment.

You need a proven prescription with plenty of backup and support in order to make the necessary changes in your lifestyle. Only then can you be assured of successful, permanent weight management.

What Makes the Snowbird Diet Different?

The Snowbird Diet is founded on the only true formula for lasting weight control. It's not a secret formula. I did not invent it. In fact, many have known its principles for years. The trouble is, very few have figured out a way to make it work in everyday life.

Most diets of recent years push one or the other of the principles, but that's like doing a jigsaw puzzle with most of the pieces missing. In fact, successful weight management is a lot like working a puzzle. All the pieces must fit perfectly with one another to complete the picture.

When someone tries to tell you that the formula for losing weight is based on funny food combinations or drinking grapefruit juice after each meal, it's a scam. If a diet doesn't fit the following formula, *it won't work*. Period.

Here is the simple, foolproof formula for *permanent* weight loss:

> BALANCED DIET
> + REGULAR AEROBIC ACTIVITY
> + STRESS MANAGEMENT
> + LIFESTYLE ADJUSTMENTS
> = PERMANENT WEIGHT LOSS

Experts Who Contributed to the Snowbird Diet

Since the Snowbird Diet is an offshoot of the program at the Southwest Bariatric Nutrition Center, it required the expertise of the top-notch professionals who have made the clinic's program so incredibly successful.

Unlike so many of today's fad diets, the Snowbird Diet has been carefully researched and developed by working professionals who are formally educated, trained, and experienced in the medical treatment of overweight.

Susan C. Olson has a Ph.D. in clinical psychology. A specialist in community psychology, group therapy, and individual therapy, she has done extensive research in reinforcement theory and behavior modification techniques. She is director of psychological services at the Southwest Bariatric Nutrition Center and is the co-author of *Keeping It Off* (Simon & Schuster, 1985), a new book on the psychology of dieting.

Jeanne Turnquist Patterson is a registered dietician, and holds a master's degree in nutrition. She is the director of Nutrition Services at the Southwest Bariatric Nutrition Center.

Karen Winden has a master's degree in exercise physiology. She is the exercise physiologist at the Southwest Bariatric Nutrition Center.

The Snowbird Diet contains the same valuable information and guidance that hundreds of people have spent thousands of dollars to obtain.

Outside the medical field, we enlisted the expertise of famed cookbook author Paula Wolfert. She served as culinary consultant for the Snowbird Diet recipes. Paula is a well-known journalist, cooking teacher, and author of three major cookbooks. Her latest cookbook, *Cooking of Southwest France*, published by Dial Press/Doubleday, has been universally praised by critics and cooks alike.

The Snowbird Diet Menus are truly exciting. My wife, Carol (who entertains at home frequently and whose cooking has been featured in *Bon Appétit* magazine) has created cuisine without equal.

Using the freshest and finest ingredients available, she has devised recipes that are simple, beautiful, and imaginative. These dishes appeal to the eye as well as the palate. Guests who are served Snowbird cuisine are always surprised that such delicious dishes can be so healthful.

Patients feel good on this diet. Many report feeling "energized." They are excited about their newfound alertness and enthusiasm, and many of them radiate a healthy glow. Is this some kind of mysterious magic? Absolutely not. It's just what happens when a person puts the formula for permanent weight loss into action.

*Patients actually **like** the diet.* Perhaps that is why they find it so easy to stick with. It's interesting. It's delicious. It's varied. It's fun. What's more, it's no trouble for the traveler or the hostess. It's simple, comfortable, and, above all, satisfying.

The Snowbird Diet lets you incorporate some of your favorites into the plan. For example, you may continue to enjoy wine, liquor, or light beer.

You don't need special supplies or equipment. All the recipes can be prepared with minimal fuss in a kitchen with ordinary equipment.

Detailed shopping lists make marketing fast and easy. You spend as little time as possible planning and thinking about meals.

You don't have to bother counting calories or carbohydrates. It's done for you.

You can enjoy food from every food group—nothing is left out.

There are simple lifestyle modifications and stress-management techniques designed to keep you enthused, positive, and excited about the program.

You will look better, not just thinner. Your eyes will be bright, your skin clear and resilient, and you will avoid that saggy look that often accompanies a major weight loss. Why? Because your body fluids will be perfectly balanced. You will be properly nourished, and you will be toning up as you lose.

If you are like most patients, you will not only look younger, you will feel younger.

The Emergency Food Plan offers alternatives. Sometimes the foods that are called for may not be available where you live or travel. So the Emergency Food Plan offers dozens of substitutions to help you follow the Snowbird Diet even under the most trying circumstances.

The Snowbird Diet Is a Diet for the 80's and Beyond

There has never been a more complete program for weight management outside an expensive private clinic.

The Snowbird Diet will help you solve the physical and emotional mysteries of weight loss forever.

It may be the most important 12 days you will ever spend.

The Snowbird Diet will be the first 12 days of a slender lifetime.

2

The Snowbird Prescription

*Weight Loss as Preventive Medicine
and Life Extension*

Having been on diets before, you may think you know all there is to know about the condition called *overweight*. Unfortunately, much of what you've been told is probably poppycock!

To set the record straight, here are some facts about overweight that will help you separate truth from fiction.

The more you understand the problem, the easier it will be to overcome it.

Why Are You Overweight?

The answer appears to be very simple. Most of you are overweight because you take in more calories than your individual metabolism needs.

Calories are units of energy.

In the body, surplus calories are stored in the form of fat.

Fat, then, is simply stored surplus energy.

Being overweight means your body has an energy glut.

For each 3,500 calories that are consumed but not burned, one pound of fat is stored.

To lose one pound of fat, you must burn off 3,500 calories.

You can do this two ways.

You can decrease the calorie input or you can increase the energy output.

The principle couldn't be simpler. But the real reasons you are overweight make the problem very complex.

Most people who suffer from a weight problem eat not because they are physiologically hungry, but because their *appetites* have been stimulated by thoughts, habits, feelings, emotions, reactions, and attitudes.

What's the Difference Between Hunger and Appetite?

In treating patients who are overweight, I have noticed many similarities in their eating habits.

For instance, the majority of these patients do not eat breakfast. They claim they're just not hungry.

While I'm not saying this is the reason they are overweight (far from it), I do think it illustrates a point.

To me, this is a classic example of how out of whack the system gets when there is an eating disorder.

You've probably always been told that you should eat a good breakfast. You may even know *why* it's important to start the day with a nourishing meal.

But did you ever stop to consider why you don't want to eat in the morning? After all, you've just gone at least eight hours without food. Your stomach is empty and you should be hungry.

Could you go eight hours without food during the day and not want to eat?

The answer is probably no.

So why don't you feel hungry at breakfast time?

The answer is simple. You have ignored your true hunger signals for so long that you are no longer tuned into them.

An overweight person eats for many reasons—but true physiological hunger is rarely among them.

Most overweight people have *learned* to eat when they are not hungry. Yet often their true hunger signals are ignored.

In a healthy person, when the body needs nourishment, the brain sends a signal that says, "I'm hungry. I need energy." The quickest way to interfere with this natural signal is to disregard it. Soon you simply stop getting the signals. Your body and mind are out of sync.

Appetite is when some feeling other than hunger tells you to eat.

Appetite, then, is *head hunger*. It can be triggered by feelings of boredom, fatigue, anger, loneliness, frustration, or even happiness.

Here's a good example of appetite at work. You have just finished a groaning holiday meal. You are uncomfortably full. Yet you can't resist eating a slice of pie. Clearly, something other than true hunger is motivating you to eat.

Here's another example. You've just had an argument with your spouse. You feel hurt and angry. Instead of dealing honestly with those feelings, you turn to food. You go on an eating binge.

You can probably think of plenty of instances when you have eaten for all the wrong reasons. Later in this book you will learn how to avoid doing that.

But for the moment, these examples merely point out the differences between hunger and appetite. *Hunger keeps you healthy. Appetite makes you fat.*

Another way to distinguish hunger from appetite is this: When you are truly hungry, almost any food will sound appetizing. But when you are having an appetite attack, you will usually crave something more akin to junk food (cookies, candy, ice cream, chips, snack foods, et cetera). An appetite attack makes nutritious foods seem less appealing.

Remember—appetite is an acquired response. It is learned behavior. And anything that is learned can be unlearned.

Before long, you'll have your own foolproof, built-in appetite suppressant. No shots, no pills, no candies. Just your own healthy body working in sync with your own healthy mind.

Is Overweight Hereditary?

There is some evidence that overweight is genetically predisposed. You may be born with the disease stamped indelibly on your chromosomes.

There is a strong chance that if your parents are overweight, you will be too. In fact, if one parent is overweight, you will have a one-in-three chance of being overweight. If both parents are overweight, your chances rise to two out of three.

Then how do we know it is not always genetic?

Because in families where one of the children is adopted, the adopted child has the same incidence of overweight as the natural children.

What does this mean?

Overweight is a condition that is learned.

And anything that is usually acquired can be unlearned.

Now that you know you don't *have* to be fat, you can go to work on the responses that have made you that way.

What's the Difference Between Obesity and Overweight?

Obesity is advanced overweight. It occurs when total body fat reaches 25 percent in men and 30 percent in women.

Obesity is a disease and a major health risk. It is associated with an alarming, lengthy list of medical complications—many of them life-threatening.

Obesity requires continuous monitoring and therapeutic treatment by a qualified physician.

Overweight usually refers to people who have fewer than 20 pounds to lose. The treatment of overweight is called "preventive" because the successful treatment of overweight prevents obesity.

Generally speaking, health risks for overweight people are not as serious as those for the obese. While a medical checkup is wise before undertaking any weight-loss plan, ongoing medical treatment for over-weight is usually not necessary.

The trouble with overweight is that if it is left untreated, it often leads to obesity. The same underlying factors bring on both conditions.

The Snowbird Diet is based on the "preventive" program at the Southwest Bariatric Nutrition Center. However, it is perfectly effective in the treatment of obesity, *provided* that the patient has regular medical checkups and remains under the care of a physician.

If you are overweight, don't let it advance to obesity. Acknowledge that obesity is the next step. Reverse your direction. Start by making a personal commitment to yourself, to your future, and to the Snowbird Diet.

If you are moderately obese, see a qualified physician before beginning the Snowbird Diet. You need therapeutic treatment now if you are to avoid further life-threatening complications. Remember, it's never too late to turn your health around. You *can* reverse accelerated aging and health deterioration. The Snowbird Diet will show you the way. For those who are severely obese and have obvious obesity-related problems, such as hypertension and diabetes, to name a few, medical monitoring is mandatory.

What Are Some of the Medical Risks Associated With Overweight?

Here is only a partial list of the many increased risks associated with overweight:

BLOOD
- High levels of triglycerides, sugar, insulin, and low-density lipoprotein (LDL, also known as the harmful cholesterol)
- Reduced levels of high-density lipoprotein (HDL, also known as good cholesterol)

BLOOD VESSELS
- One pound of extra fat adds 200 miles of blood vessels to your body
- Inflammation of the veins

CARDIOVASCULAR SYSTEM
Heart
- High blood pressure
- Higher resting heart rate
- Enlarged heart
- Arrhythmias (irregular heartbeats)
- Heart failure
- Hypertension

MAJOR ORGANS
Brain
- Stroke
- Cerebral hemorrhage

Lungs
- Respiratory distress due to shallow breathing
- Sleep apnea

Stomach
- Cancer

Liver
- Cancer
- Cirrhosis
- Hepatobiliary disease

Pancreas
- Cancer

Kidneys
- Renal disease
- Hypertension

Gallbladder
- Cancer
- Gallstones

Colon
- Cancer
- Decreased intestinal mobility

Uterus and Ovaries
- Cancer
- Irregular menstrual cycles
- Heavy menstrual flow
- Reduced reproductive capacity

SKIN
- Skin ulcers
- Skin irritations
- Increased facial hair

MUSCLES AND CELLS
- Reduced insulin sensitivity
- Diabetes

SKELETAL SYSTEM
- Lower-back problems
- Ruptured discs
- Degenerative joint disease
- Gout
- Acute arthritis and inflammation of the joints

OTHER RISKS
- Excessive fluid retention
- Susceptibility to infections
- Decreased sex drive
- Hernias
- Greater risk in surgery
- Psychological problems

Can Health Problems That Accompany Overweight Be Cured?

The human body, being the miraculous mechanism that it is, can recover from almost all obesity-related health problems when the formula for permanent weight loss is practiced.
Remember:

BALANCED DIET
+ REGULAR AEROBIC ACTIVITIES
+ STRESS MANAGEMENT
+ LIFESTYLE ADJUSTMENTS
= PERMANENT WEIGHT LOSS

When this formula is incorporated into your life, your body can begin to return to health almost immediately.

At the Southwest Bariatric Nutrition Center there is equipment to help gauge the cardiovascular physiological age of each patient. When patients start the program, they are tested to see how old their bodies really are, regardless of chronological age. Generally, the patients who are obese test out to be much older physiologically than their actual chronological ages.

However, when they complete the program, most of these patients' test results show a startling improvement. Almost all have returned to a physical condition equal to or better than that of people of their own chronological age.

The metabolic flow sheet (see illustration on pages 24–25) is a visual example of such a case.

When the patient R.L. came to the Southwest Bariatric Nutrition Center, he was 41 years old. Yet his coronary risk factors were those of a man much older. R.L. was morbidly obese—170 pounds overweight.

When we determine one very important risk factor of a patient, we divide his total cholesterol count by the amount of good cholesterol (HDL) he has. Total cholesterol is actually composed of two types of cholesterol—"bad" (low-density lipoprotein) and "good" (high-density lipoprotein).

LDL, the bad cholesterol, is thought to be responsible for "clogging" the arteries. It results from unhealthful living habits and poor dietary intake.

HDL, the good cholesterol, seems to help keep the arteries unobstructed—like a drain cleaner. It is manufactured naturally by the body to control too much LDL, and is enhanced by exercise.

When you are overweight and suffering from the effects of an unhealthful lifestyle (poor diet, no exercise, and uncontrolled stress) LDL becomes elevated and HDL declines.

Triglycerides (fats in the blood) may be elevated when you eat too much starch and sugar.

In the case of R.L., our 41-year-old patient, his LDL was high, his HDL was low, his triglycerides were high, and his overall cholesterol was high, making his coronary risk factors nothing short of dangerous.

Instead of being a healthful, vital, exuberant young man, he had taken on the ills and outlook of someone much older.

After nine months of treatment at the Southwest Bariatric Nutrition Center, R.L.'s weight was down 165 pounds. His physical appearance and mental outlook had improved dramatically.

His physiological age had dropped to below that of his actual years. His coronary risk factors were now better than normal for a man his age.

It's Never Too Late

If you are on the road to obesity and its related medical problems, it is important to know that simple changes in your diet and lifestyle can reverse the process. They can set you on the road to a lifetime of physical and mental well-being.

It's not too late. You can recover your health, improve your outlook, and be the vital, energetic human being you were meant to be. It is much easier and cheaper to maintain good health than to regain it once it is lost.

Of course, no treatment in the world can measure up to the prevention of a disease in the first place.

The Snowbird Diet Is Preventive Medicine at Its Best

With the cost of health care soaring and no ceiling in sight, I continue to emphasize the critical importance of *preventive medicine*.

In medical school, we are trained to treat the illness, and too often not to prevent it.

Preventing illness is usually out of the doctor's hands anyway. Most of our patients come to see us after the damage has been done. They wait until there is a major problem before they seek help. By then it's too late for preventive tactics.

According to the Department of Health, the cost of medical care in 1950 was between $10 billion and $12 billion.

Twenty years later it was $60 billion to $70 billion.

In 1980 the cost was a staggering $250 billion.

In another twenty years the cost of medical care may be out of the reach of many, many people if this trend continues.

If the treatment of disease is too expensive, what is the answer?

Preventive Medicine

In 1982, 160,000 coronary bypass operations were done in the United States at a total cost of nearly $4 billion. We know that heart disease

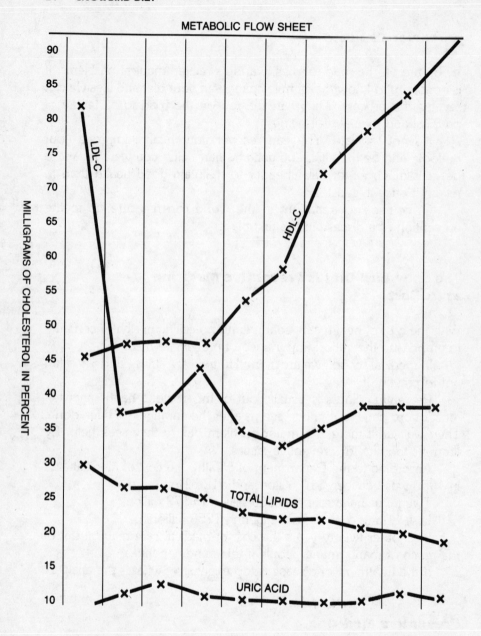

METABOLIC FLOW SHEET

This metabolic flow sheet shows the dramatic reduction in the coronary risk factors of R.L., a patient at the Southwest Bariatric Nutrition Center who lost 165 pounds.

As his weight declined, his LDL (bad cholesterol) was reduced and his HDL (good cholesterol) was boosted. After the weight loss, R.L.'s cholesterol/HDL risk factor fell from a dangerous 5 to a safe, comfortable 2—below normal for a man his age.

His triglycerides and combined cholesterol count also dropped markedly.

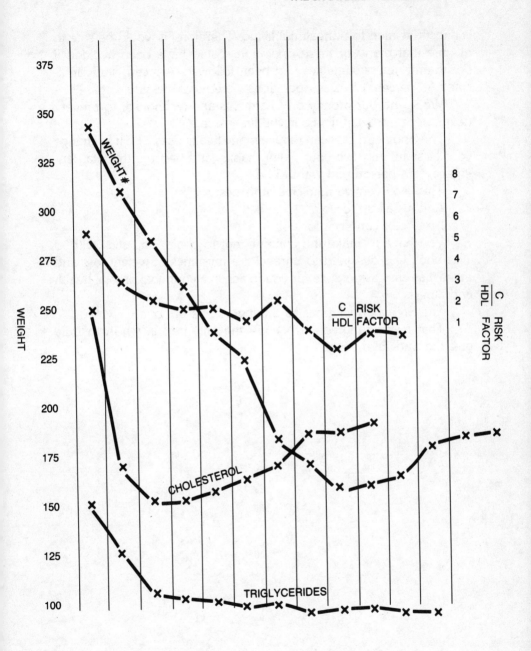

is directly related to unhealthful living. Therefore, it would be safe to assume that many of these operations could have been avoided if health and fitness strategies had been followed. A recent study indicated 60 percent of these operations were not necessary.

We spend our money on treatments and technology to prevent death, not to prevent illness in the first place.

The Snowbird Diet can reduce many health risks. Use it to change your lifestyle, improve your eating habits, and become the vital, energetic, trim person you want to be.

This is preventive medicine at its best.

And it's all up to you.

No doctor can do it for you.

You have to make the commitment to health and stick with it. This book was designed to unravel the mysteries of weight loss and make it as easy as possible for you to achieve your goal of total health and fitness.

The Snowbird Diet has all the ingredients but one.

That missing ingredient is you—the only person who can truly give the Snowbird wings.

3

Set Yourself Up for Success

Many dieters are so impatient to start losing weight that they jump the gun and plunge into a diet before they are really prepared.

Here are some of the most common mistakes they make: They start a diet

a. without fully reading or understanding what it is all about
b. before they have "goof-proofed" their surroundings
c. without having the proper supplies on hand
d. before they've made a total commitment to the diet

As I mentioned earlier, the Snowbird Diet is composed of many parts. Each must work in concert with the others if the program is to have permanent results.

Before You Begin the Snowbird Diet

First things first. *Read the entire book from cover to cover.* Don't start the diet until you understand each and every part of it.

If you have questions, reread specific chapters or refer to "Snowbird Dieters Ask the Doctor" at the back of the book.

As you read the book, make notes on any special supplies or equipment you may need to buy. Don't begin the diet until you have purchased everything you need for it. There are very few requirements, but they are vital to the diet.

Goof-Proof Your Surroundings

Most people are overweight because they have learned bad habits. In order to break the fat cycle, you will have to be scrupulously honest with yourself.

Do you have snacks tucked away in "secret" places?

Do you always keep a supply of fattening foods on hand "in case of emergency" and then eat them during snack attacks?

Are there ingredients in your home or office that let you whip up a fattening snack on a moment's impulse?

Do you buy fattening foods for other members of the family and then snack on them yourself?

Do you keep high-calorie snacks in your car or at work?

Do you often snack with your head in the refrigerator?

Do you snack in the car on the way home from the grocery store?

Do you have special stops along regular travel routes where you buy fattening foods (a doughnut shop, an ice-cream parlor, a cookie store, et cetera)?

Do certain activities seem to compel you to eat fattening foods? For instance, when you go to the movies, must you have popcorn? When you watch television, must you drink beer or nibble on salted nuts?

Do you cruise the supermarket aisles looking for snack ideas?

Do you cook or bake fattening snacks for others as an excuse to munch on them yourself?

If someone gives you a fattening-food gift, do you feel compelled to eat it?

Do you frequent restaurants that serve foods you can't resist?

Do you read magazines with recipes or food ads that seem to fire up your appetite?

When you see food commercials on television, do you automatically reach for a snack?

If you have been completely honest, you will probably have answered yes to many of these questions.

That doesn't mean you're a bad person. Nor does it mean you are hopelessly weak-willed. I'll tell you a little secret about willpower. *Nobody* is automatically equipped with it. It must be developed. And the only way to develop your self-control is to begin to make *conscious* choices.

It's quite possible that all the snacking you have been doing is *subconscious*. In other words, you've been doing the same things over and over for so long that they are now automatic; you don't even have to think about them. The Snowbird Diet will teach you how to break out of these destructive habits a little at a time.

First things first. **Before** you start this diet, you must **goof-proof** your surroundings.

Go through your house or office with a fine-tooth comb. Remove all the snack foods from the refrigerator, the car, the desk, the pantry, the cupboards, under the bed—wherever you have put them. Empty the candy dishes and cookie jars. Be thorough and honest. Only you know where temptation lurks. Gather up all those fattening snacks and get rid of them! Throw them into the trash. They'll look a lot better in the garbage than on your hips.

From now on, if there are no snacks around, you won't be tempted to eat them.

Begin to alter your lifestyle to avoid the things that lead to fat.

If you pass tempting snack spots during the regular course of your day, change your route. Avoid going past the ice-cream parlor or the doughnut shop.

Don't keep fattening snacks on hand for the family, either. Let them benefit from your new commitment to fitness as well.

If certain activities trigger your desire for food (such as popcorn at the movies), avoid those activities for a while, or think of better ways to handle them. You may find that taking a healthful munchie to the movies will placate your urge to eat without wrecking your diet.

Don't torture yourself by reading recipes or watching food commercials on TV. Give away food magazines or cancel subscriptions. Don't even crack a cookbook unless it's one devoted to light, healthful eating. When a food commercial comes on TV, leave the room. Sip a cold, no-calorie carbonated beverage until the urge to eat has passed.

You might be thinking, "Isn't this a lot of trouble to go through just to get ready for a diet?"

To that we say: Anything worth doing is worth doing right. The only way to get rid of the fat that makes you unhappy is to devote yourself to becoming slender. It will take effort.

But in the end, can you think of a more worthwhile endeavor?

So for now, out of sight, smell, and thought means out of mind. Goof-proof your surroundings *now* so that you won't be tempted in a moment of weakness later.

This is a major step toward committing yourself 100 percent to success.

Buy All the Equipment and Ingredients You Will Need

Before you begin the Snowbird Diet, it is mandatory that you obtain the required food and equipment.

Going on the Snowbird Diet is like going on an expedition. You wouldn't dream of embarking on an adventure without first assembling the proper supplies to ensure a successful journey.

While the Snowbird Diet demands very little in the way of supplies, the few things that are specified are extremely important. In addition to specific foods and beverages, you will need a spiral notebook and perhaps proper play clothes (all are explained in detail later). A heavy-duty, non-stick skillet with a lid is a good investment, too. I recommend T-Fal brand, but any well-made skillet will do.

As you go through this book, make careful notes on what you will need to buy. Detailed food shopping lists are given to help make the task of marketing easier and less time-consuming.

Buy *everything* you need *before* you begin the diet.

This initial investment of time, effort, and money is vital for two reasons.

One: It is the *only* way to start the Snowbird Diet on the right foot. If you begin before you have the proper supplies, your expedition will have a much smaller chance of success.

Two: Making an investment of time, effort, and money is the first tangible proof of your commitment toward the goal of a slender lifetime. It will prepare you psychologically for the success that is to come.

Make a Strong, Positive Commitment to Think Thin

Make a decision to devote yourself to the Snowbird Diet and stick with it. Period. Don't allow pessimism to creep into your head. You'll have to be constantly on guard against nasty negatives—they are firmly entrenched in your thoughts or you wouldn't be overweight.

Most people who are overweight are plagued with negative thoughts, or *fat think*. Before you start the Snowbird Diet, eliminate fat think. Don't say "I *guess* I'll *try* this new diet," or, "I'll give it a whirl, but it probably won't work," or, "I'll try it out, but it's probably too hard."

Instead, state your intentions in bold, enthusiastic positives: "This is a good diet. I will lose weight. I will look better. I will feel better. I will be happy."

If you don't believe these words, start repeating them to yourself throughout the day. Before you get up in the morning, while you are driving to work, during quiet moments, and before you go to sleep at night, repeat:

This is a good diet. I will lose weight. I will look better. I will feel better. I will be happy.

Make the commitment to *yourself*. You must want to be slender for *you*, not because someone else wants you to lose weight.

But don't sit around waiting for the motivation to strike you. Get up and make your own motivation. Actively think thin. Repeat: **This is a good diet. I will lose weight. I will look better. I will feel better. I will be happy.**

Whether you know it or not, you have just taken a giant step toward becoming the slender person you want to be.

That giant step is toward a positive attitude.

It will spur motivation and help you over the rough spots. Repeat it, repeat it, repeat it. It will become just as automatic as your old fat think.

Keeping a Snowbird Workbook

What? A workbook? It sounds like grammar school! Well, in a sense it is. Remember we told you that being fat is a *learned behavior*? Being slender is also a *learned behavior*. The Snowbird Workbook will help you learn how to be slender and stay that way.

The workbook is an essential element in the Snowbird Diet and one that many patients enjoy. It helps you to focus clearly on goals— to see where you're going and where you've been.

Select a notebook that you like. Choose one in a size that's comfortable for reading, writing, and carrying. Generally, a tiny notebook is too restricting, while a large one may be too cumbersome.

A plain spiral notebook of medium size with lined pages works very well, but if you'd rather have a leather-bound volume with blank pages, be my guest.

The point is, *you* will be using the Snowbird Workbook for several weeks to come. Choose something *you* can live with.

The Snowbird Workbook will function as a companion to *The Snowbird Diet* book. You will be taking it almost everywhere you go. In it you will establish fitness goals, chart progress, learn techniques for self-awareness, and plan for success.

You will use the Snowbird Workbook throughout the 12-Day Diet and well into the maintenance program. Many patients continue to keep a workbook indefinitely. It serves as a reference, a guide, an inspiration, a record, and a personal diary.

PART II

How the Snowbird
Diet Works

4

Wondrous Water
One of the Secrets to
Successful Weight Loss

For years people have sought a magical cure for fat. Thousands of different diets have appeared, each claiming to have the answer. Fantastic concoctions have been marketed by the truckload, though pitifully few have offered any real hope of lasting weight loss. Herbal wraps, tonics, syrups, injections, tablets, capsules, candies, sweatsuits, steam cabinets, and exotic fruit combinations. You name it, somebody's tried it.

Ironically, the only true "magic potion" for permanent weight loss has been largely ignored. I'm talking about H_2O. That's right. The ordinary stuff that flows out of your faucet for free. Most of us take it for granted. We continually pass it up for beverages brewed, bottled, or bubbly.

Incredible as it may seem, water is quite possibly the single most important catalyst in losing weight and keeping it off.

Here are some startling—yet scientific—facts about the benefits of water to weight loss:

- *Water can help your body metabolize fat.*
- *Water can eliminate fluid retention.*
- *Water can help you lose all the weight you want and keep it off for good.*

Throw away your diuretics, toss the laxatives, flush the appetite suppressants. Water does all these jobs better, yet it's safe, natural, and healthful.

Water works—if you learn how to use it.

THE LIQUID OF LIFE

Life without water would last about 7 days. Every form of life on earth depends on water.

Adequate water is essential for the human body to perform at its peak. Like the earth, the human body is 70 percent water. A loss of 10 percent body water would be critical. More than that might prove fatal.

Where Does the Body Get the Water It Needs?

About half comes from beverages we drink—water, tea, coffee, soft drinks, milk, beer, wine, et cetera.

A small portion is *metabolic water*—water we manufacture as we metabolize food.

The rest comes from food. Meat, for instance, is 70 percent water. Fruits can be up to 90 percent water. Even bread is 20 percent water.

How Does the Body Use Water?

All reactions in the body take place in water. It's the catalyst for enzymatic reactions.

Blood plasma, which is 90 percent water, can be called the body's main waterway. Food is transported to cells. Waste is carried away, passed through the kidneys and out in the urine. About half our fluid intake is expelled this way.

Water makes breathing possible. It moistens the harsh, dry air. We exhale about 20 percent of our water intake.

The digestive system uses several *gallons* of water daily to process food. Digestive enzymes are made almost entirely of water.

The body uses water in its cooling system. When it gets to be 92 degrees F. outside, or when we exercise briskly, the body heats up. This heat must be dissipated. So the body pumps moisture through the muscles to the skin, where it evaporates and cools down the system.

Where Does the Body Store Water?

Water input must equal water output. Furthermore, water distribution throughout the body must be balanced. The body continually strives to maintain *water balance.*

Half our water is stored in the cells (intracellular).

The rest is stored outside the cells (extracellular), which includes fluid between cells and plasma inside blood vessels.

If Lean Body Mass Is 70 Percent Water, What's the Other 30 Percent?

Muscle, organ tissue, and fat. Only 3 percent of this fat is essential. It is found in and around most vital organs such as the kidneys and gastrointestinal tract.

The rest of the stored fat is the stuff that won't fit into the clothes we want to wear.

The bad news for women is, they store more fat than men do because of different hormone levels.

Water and Weight Loss

By now it's clear that water is vital for the human body to run in top form. But how can water help you lose weight?

Water Suppresses the Appetite Naturally.

Water Helps the Body Metabolize Stored Fat.

Studies have shown that a decrease in water intake will cause fat deposits to increase, while an increase in water intake can actually reduce fat deposits.

In other words, *drinking water can help rid your body of stored fat.*

Here's how it works. The kidneys can't function properly without enough water. When they don't work up to capacity, some of their load is dumped onto the liver.

One of the liver's primary functions is to metabolize stored fat. The liver turns this fat into usable energy for the body.

If the liver has to do some of the kidneys' work, it can't operate at full throttle. Therefore, it metabolizes less fat. More fat remains stored in the body and weight loss stops.

What could be worse for the dieter!

Drinking Adequate Water Is the Best Treatment for Fluid Retention.

Sound crazy? It's the most sensible solution to water retention you'll ever find!

When an otherwise healthy person has a problem with water retention, he usually does two things: he drinks *less* water and/or starts taking diuretics.

These are the worst possible things to do.

First, when the body gets less water, it perceives this as a threat to survival. To conserve what it has, it begins to hold on to every drop. Water is stored in *extracellular* spaces (outside the cells). This shows up as swollen feet, legs, hands, and so on.

Diuretics are a temporary solution at best. They only mask the real problem. The diuretic forces out stored water, along with some essential nutrients. Again, the body perceives a threat and will replace the lost water at the first opportunity. Thus, the condition returns almost immediately.

What happens? The person usually graduates to progressively stronger diuretics, which can eventually lead to a dependency. Worst of all, the problem of water retention goes unsolved.

The Overweight Person Needs More Water Than a Thin Person.

The larger a person is, the larger his *metabolic load*. He needs to process more fuel to keep going—just as a big sedan needs more fuel than a small sports car. Since we know that water is the key to fat metabolism, it follows that the overweight person needs more water.

This is why so many overweight people retain water. Their bodies get too little water, so their systems hang on to what they get. The only way to overcome this problem is to give the body what it needs to function—plenty of water. Only in this way will stored water be released.

Water Helps to Maintain Proper Muscle Tone.

It gives muscles their natural ability to contract and it keeps them from becoming dehydrated.

Water Prevents the Sagging Skin That Usually Follows Weight Loss.

Shrinking cells are buoyed by water, which plumps the skin and leaves it clear, healthy, and resilient.

Water Helps Rid the Body of Waste.

During weight loss, the body has a lot more waste to get rid of. All that metabolized fat must be shed. Again, to ease the load on the kidneys, adequate water helps flush out the waste.

Water Can Help Relieve Constipation.

When the body gets too little water, it siphons water from internal sources. The colon is one primary source. Result? Constipation. The feces become hard and dry.

Constipation is too often treated with laxatives. Aside from leading to a dependency, this solution never addresses the root of the problem.

The whole miserable cycle can be avoided. When a person drinks the correct amount of water, normal bowel function usually returns.

Sodium and Common Sense

On this subject many diet gurus launch into what I call their "sodium scare sermon."

Salt may be a four-letter word, but it's not a *dirty* word.

This is not to say that you should run out and stock up on pretzels and anchovies. Rather, let common sense be your guide.

Someone once said, "The trouble with common sense is that it is so uncommon." I believe you can't exercise common sense unless you have the facts. So here are the facts about sodium.

How Much Salt Does Your Body Need?

Medically, it's thought that 500 to 2,000 mg. (¼ to 1 teaspoon) per day is enough to maintain good health.

The average American diet contains ten to twelve times this amount. That's where the trouble lies. Salt is not necessarily sinister in *moderation*. But *excess* salt can lead to problems for people who are "salt sensitive." About 20 percent of the population is salt sensitive. This means they have an adverse reaction to anything but a minimal amount of salt. Of these people, about 12 percent may develop high blood pressure.

Is High Blood Pressure Related to Salt Intake?

The volume of blood can increase and the walls of the blood vessels can be constricted as a result of excess sodium intake. However, recent research seems to indicate that too much sodium may not be as guilty as too *little* potassium and calcium.

Does Excess Salt Contribute to Water Retention?

It can. Your body will tolerate sodium only in a certain concentration. The more salt you eat, the more water your system retains to dilute it to a safe solution.

Salt intake makes you thirsty. This releases an *antidiuretic hormone* that causes water to be retained. The water is packed away in extracellular spaces that expand. This means swollen hands, feet, legs, and so on.

For your kidneys to expel the excess sodium, they need more

water. If you don't drink enough, the water will automatically be siphoned from internal sources.

It's the same old story—the body's way of coping with too little water is to store up what it has.

How Do You Get Rid of Excess Sodium?

Drink more water. It's that simple. Water is forced through the kidneys, taking the excess sodium with it.

In addition, the body has some natural checks and balances for dealing with sodium. Eat no salt, and the body secretes a hormone called *aldosterone* to hang on to the sodium it needs. Eat a little salt, and the aldosterone level drops. Eat too much salt, and extracellular spaces begin to expand with stored water. When this happens, another hormone is released to prompt the loss of both the excess sodium and the water.

All these checks and balances work in concert to help maintain perfect water balance.

But none of them will work without an ample supply of water.

What Are Some Other Causes of Water Retention?

Besides excess sodium and too little water, there are many other causes—some of which require you to be under a physician's care.

- Failure of the heart to pump blood adequately
- Chronic protein deficiency (possibly caused by kidney disease)
- Hormone imbalance due to birth-control pills or the menstrual cycle
- Abnormally high refined-carbohydrate intake, which can induce an antidiuretic-hormone effect
- Emotional upset can also release an antidiuretic hormone
- Local causes, like *thrombophlebitis* (blood clots in the veins); *lipedema* (blockage of the fluid outside the veins); or *lipemia* (fats blocking return blood flow in the legs)
- Drugs such as blood-pressure medications, cortisone, arthritis medications, and many, many others

Do Some People Need More Salt Than Others?

Yes. People living in hot, dry climates or those who do strenuous work or exercise need more sodium and more water. It is my feeling that at least 50 percent of the people living in the arid Southwest are somewhat dehydrated. This means they could be physically, mentally, and emotionally below par.

Studies show that a person doing normal daily activities in very hot, dry weather can lose as much as 1 quart of water *per hour*. Those doing heavy work or strenuous exercise can lose 2 quarts or more an hour! They also lose vital sodium. When the sodium level drops too much, blood pressure also drops. The symptoms are weakness, fatigue, dizziness, and faintness.

For a quick pick-me-up, I tell patients to drink a cup of beef bouillon or consommé. I don't recommend chicken bouillon because it's not high enough in sodium.

Should You Ever Take Salt Tablets?

Absolutely not! They force water out of extracellular spaces and into the stomach. This draws water away from the muscles and skin, where it's needed to cool the body. Beef bouillon is a much better solution.

How Can One Avoid Eating Too Much Sodium?

You don't have to go on a rigid salt-free diet. Instead, just be aware of the products that are high in salt: processed wheat and bran flakes, most canned foods, bacon, ham, salted fish, processed cheeses, most snack foods, and foods with additives like mono*sodium* glutamate. Read labels. Most manufacturers are required to list the amounts of sodium their products contain.

Foods naturally low in salt are fruits, fruit juices, fresh vegetables, and generally anything you cook from scratch, because you can add little or none.

How to Drink Water and Lose Weight

We've discovered some remarkable truths about the role water plays in weight control.

1. *The body will not function properly without enough water.* Thus, it can't metabolize stored fat efficiently.
2. *Retained water shows up as excess weight on your scale.* Or, as I tell my patients, "A pint is a pound the world around."
3. *To get rid of excess water you must drink more water.*
4. *Drinking water is* **essential** *to weight loss.*

How Much Water Is Enough?

On the average, a person should drink 8 (8-ounce) glasses every day. That's about 2 quarts. However, the overweight person needs 1 additional glass for *every* 25 pounds of excess weight. The amount you drink also should be increased if you exercise briskly or if the weather is hot and dry.

Snowbird Dieters should drink a *minimum* of 2 quarts per day.

Will You Have to Move into the Bathroom?

Not *if* you drink as prescribed. Follow this schedule:
Morning:　1 quart consumed over a period of 30 minutes.
Noon:　1 quart consumed over a period of 30 minutes.
Evening:　1 quart consumed between five and six o'clock.

The Drinking Schedule Is Important

It's important to follow the drinking schedule, for more reasons than one.

A patient of mine went out shopping all day and didn't drink a drop of water until she got home late that evening. Then she drank 5 quarts of water before going to bed. No, she was not up all night. In fact, the opposite was true.

The minute she went to bed, her body secreted its normal anti-diuretic hormone. It put a lock on all that water.

The next day, she weighed in 10 pounds heavier!

Over the next two days the water was slowly released, but she learned the value of drinking water as prescribed.

The Breakthrough Point

When the body gets the water it needs to function optimally, its fluids are perfectly balanced.

When this happens you have reached the "breakthrough point," so named by well-known California physician and bariatrician Peter Lindner, M.D.

What does this mean?

- Endocrine-gland function improves.
- Fluid retention is alleviated because stored water is lost.
- More fat is used as fuel because the liver is free to metabolize stored fat.
- Natural thirst returns.
- There is a loss of hunger almost overnight.

After you reach the breakthrough point you won't have to force yourself to drink the proper amount of water. You will *want* to drink it.

What Happens If You Stop Drinking Enough Water?

Your body fluids will be thrown out of balance again. You'll have to go back and force another "breakthrough."

What Happens When You're "Out of Balance"?

You'll experience

1. fluid retention
2. unexplained weight gain
3. loss of thirst

At What Temperature Should the Water Be?

Cold is better. Cold water is absorbed into the system more quickly than warm water. And some evidence suggests that drinking cold water can actually help burn calories.

Is Water the Only Liquid You Can Drink?

Coffee, tea, and diet soft drinks should be taken only in moderation. Have no more than 2 cups of coffee or tea a day. Limit soft drinks to 2 per day. These beverages have an adverse effect on weight loss. Eliminate them completely if you can, since caffeinated drinks (coffee, tea, diet colas) stimulate the appetite. However, if you now drink large amounts of caffeinated beverages, it might be wise to cut down slowly. Cold-turkey caffeine withdrawal can trigger severe headaches.

Are Decaffeinated Drinks Okay?

In moderation. Most still contain a degree of caffeine. And decaffeinated sodas may also contain excessive amounts of sodium, so read the labels.

Diet Drinks Are Not for Dieters!

Most so-called diet drinks are loaded with sodium, which we know can cause fluid retention. This shows up as added pounds on the scale.

The high levels of phosphates in diet drinks interfere with the body's absorption of calcium, which can also be critical to the dieter.

What About Bottled Mineral Waters?

They're fine. But how many of us can drink 3 quarts of Perrier a day? Why not save them for special occasions—to sip instead of a cocktail. They're delicious with a squirt of fresh lime or lemon or with a dash of bitters. Salt-free varieties are now available.

What If Tap Water Has an Unpleasant Taste?

Buy bottled water. If that's not convenient, try chilling the tap water thoroughly, with a few thin slices of lemon added to the pitcher. One lemon slice to a glass of plain water gives it a nice fresh flavor. This works well for travelers who may run into unpleasant-tasting water. A fresh lemon is easy to carry with you.

5

Another Snowbird Secret:

Lower Blood Insulin and Weight Loss

The Snowbird Diet is based on the very latest medical research and clinical experience. In working to unravel the mysteries of obesity, a hormone called *insulin* has become the focus of many studies. We now believe that insulin plays an important role in obesity.

For instance, research indicates that the level of blood insulin may explain why some people can eat a mountain of food and not gain an ounce, while others continue to gain even on severely restricted diets.

All research seems to lead to one surprising conclusion: Counting calories may not necessarily ensure weight loss. If the blood insulin is high, the body *cannot* metabolize fat efficiently.

The Snowbird Diet has been designed to reduce blood-insulin levels so that weight loss will be maximized.

What Is Insulin?

Insulin is a hormone secreted by a gland called the pancreas.

Insulin makes it possible for food (in the form of blood glucose) to enter the cells and be converted into energy.

Normally, the pancreas produces just the right amount of insulin for the job. Cells respond as they should and blood glucose is burned as fuel. When this mechanism does not function properly, instead of being converted to energy, blood glucose is converted to fat.

How Does Insulin Affect the Dieter?

Studies have shown that most people who are obese do not have normal insulin-cell-food mechanisms. Obesity brings on a condition called *hyperinsulinemia*. In other words, obesity raises the level of blood insulin.

This condition can be a critical factor in weight loss. It appears that high blood insulin can actually *prevent* weight loss. Worse, it might even force weight gain even if the caloric intake is severely restricted.

This explains why some people continue to gain weight even on very low-calorie diets.

How Does High Blood Insulin Interfere with Weight Loss?

When the insulin level is high, as it is in many who are obese, as much as 50 percent of the food eaten can be automatically converted to fat.

Hyperinsulinemia causes fat to be built up rather than burned off.

If you have high blood insulin, even if you go on a 500-calorie-a-day diet, you could conceivably *gain weight*. A high blood-insulin level might turn at least half of what you eat directly into fat.

Some people are affected more adversely than others. There is no way to predict who has or will develop significant hyperinsulinemia.

What Can Be Done to Correct High Blood Insulin?

The Snowbird Diet combats hyperinsulinemia.

The foods were carefully selected and balanced so that the protein-to-carbohydrate ratio will not only reduce blood insulin but will promote quicker weight loss as well. Your body will be better able to metabolize fat.

Even though you will consume around 800–1000 calories per day on the Snowbird Diet, the combination of foods will ensure fat loss at the maximum possible rate.

How Does the Snowbird Diet Reduce High Blood Insulin?

For one thing, it restricts the intake of simple carbohydrates.

Simple carbohydrates, such as highly refined white flour and sugar (and all the products made with these ingredients), are the real culprits. Cookies, cakes, most baked goods, ice cream, and many packaged and processed foods contain simple carbohydrates.

Because of their adverse effect on weight loss, these foods are often referred to as "fat glue." They boost the insulin level, which in turn prevents the proper metabolization of blood glucose and keeps fat "glued" to the cells.

Let's say you are on an 800-calorie-a-day diet. In theory, you should lose weight very quickly. But if simple carbohydrates are part of your intake, weight loss could be slowed or even stopped. Any lopsided ratio of simple carbohydrates to protein will kick up your blood-insulin level and you might even gain weight.

In order to metabolize fat efficiently, you must eat a diet that lowers blood insulin. The Snowbird Diet is designed to do this. It can be a very effective treatment for hyperinsulinemia in people who are overweight.

Controlling blood insulin is just one of the many elements that work to make the Snowbird Diet a comprehensive weight-management plan.

Note: Recent research from a major hypertension clinic has indicated that high insulin levels are also responsible for high blood pressure in obese patients. When the insulin drops to normal by controlling carbohydrates, there is a dramatic drop in blood pressure in most (90 percent of all) patients.

6

The Snowbird Diet

Menus and Magic for
12 Slenderizing Days

I f you've had your fill of unappetizing, so-called diet food, then you
are in for a real treat. The Snowbird Diet is unlike any diet you've
ever tried. While so many diets offer food that is bland, boring,
and monotonous, the Snowbird Diet serves up menus that are so
delicious and interesting, you may forget you're on a diet.

At the Southwest Bariatric Nutrition Center, we don't believe that
losing weight should mean giving up the enjoyment of food. Far from
it. In fact, it's been our experience that people who genuinely enjoy
the food on a diet are more likely to succeed because they don't feel
deprived.

The Snowbird Diet is a gastronomic adventure. It destroys the
myth once and for all that slenderizing food has to be humdrum and
glum.

My wife, Carol, who is the executive director of the Southwest
Bariatric Nutrition Center and a celebrated cook as well, has developed, with ideas from Paula Wolfert, the menus and recipes you are
about to discover. Her dishes have received rave reviews from guests
and professional cooks alike. Within the confines of strict dietary daily
allowances formulated by dietician Jeanne Patterson, R.D., Carol has
developed menus for meals that are not only beautifully prepared but
uncommonly delicious as well.

This chapter, with its menus, recipes, and expertise on food, was written by my wife. She is undoubtedly the culinary master of this team.

Carol's Comments

As the wife of the director of a total wellness program, it has been my project for the last seven years to prove that "diet" food can be delicious. I set out to create cuisine that could be enjoyed and served with pride without letting guests know that the food was low in calories.

Amazingly, most of our dinner guests never guessed. I'm amused when I think of the times people have said, "Carol, this food is so delicious. How do you stay so slim cooking this way?"

I have always loved to cook and to entertain lavishly. I adore good food. Being married to a weight-management specialist might well have been a culinary straitjacket for me, but I was not about to let that happen. After years of cooking classes and food experimentation, I have found that making calorie-conscious cuisine is the most refined, creative, and challenging kind of cooking there is!

In low-calorie cooking, you can't rely on many of the classic cooking props that have been used over the years. Heavy sauces, lots of sugar and salt, gobs of butter and oil—none of these can be used to hide the flavors of less-than-perfect ingredients. But once you throw off the shackles of yesterday's cooking dictates, you begin to discover the subtle, delicate flavors of fresh, fine-quality food that has been carefully prepared.

When you start with the finest ingredients and cook them to perfection, all those fattening extras are totally unnecessary.

Improving Your Palate

When you are accustomed to eating too much sugar, salt, and fat, your taste buds are desensitized to more interesting, subtle flavors.

One goal of the Snowbird Diet is to reduce the amounts of sugar, salt, and fat in your cooking to let you acquire new taste and appreciation for finer foods.

Salt is not eliminated. A little salt is not harmful and it also enhances the flavor of food. Too much salt, however, not only masks natural goodness, it hides rancidity.*

Refined sugar (and flour) acts as fat glue by keeping fat stuck to the cells. It is a villain in any weight-loss plan. If you find your sweet tooth hard to shake at first, use a no-calorie sweetener. Remember, though, the goal is to cleanse your palate of the taste for exaggerated sweetness. You must learn to savor the honest taste of food, not hide it with cloying sweetener.

The Snowbird Diet uses fats and oils very carefully. Like salt, in small amounts they are not harmful, and they do add a flavorful dimension to many dishes.

You are about to acquire a new appreciation of truly fine food. This is not just temporary. This new awareness will enhance your enjoyment of good food for the rest of your life.

Learning to Eat Less and Enjoy It More

Many of our patients have complained that past diets have left them feeling deprived. So many of their favorite foods were forbidden that they were constantly yearning for something. That nagging feeling of deprivation is downright dangerous to the dieter. It leads to binging and weight gain.

With the Snowbird Diet, you will learn how to eat less, but enjoy it a lot more. You probably already know that overeating isn't satisfying. Here's proof: How many times have you overeaten, only to continue to want something else? The real pleasure in food does not lie in the quantity consumed.

The Snowbird Diet stresses quality over quantity. You won't be hungry—there's plenty of food. But we don't believe in filling you up with tasteless low-calorie snacks as some diets do. Instead, we provide healthy portions of delicious, interesting foods that will provide a total dining experience. You won't be mindlessly swallowing bland, boring food—you will be experiencing the joy of fine dining.

The Snowbird menus have been carefully planned to provide exciting contrasts in color, texture, and taste. We know that the en-

---

*If you have high blood pressure, or have a history of heart disease in your family, consult with your doctor before beginning the Snowbird Diet.

joyment of eating is often greater when the food is attractive and beautifully served.

Pleasurable eating comes from deliberately savoring good food, having an abundant variety, enjoying fine quality, and seasoning food in such a way that the flavor is heightened and enhanced, not masked or spoiled.

Enjoying a Meal the Snowbird Way

When you get into the habit of eating too much, you are likely to eat quickly and carelessly. As a result, you gulp down platefuls of food without even realizing it. You feel full, but you don't feel satisfied.

Once you learn how, enjoying a flavorful meal can be a pure sensual pleasure.

The first thing to remember is to eat slowly. You can make a meal (one plate of food) last for hours if you like. Savor and mentally record every bite. My husband sometimes recommends that patients switch from a knife and fork to chopsticks for a while to slow down their eating. The important thing to remember is to be aware of each bite you put into your mouth. Chew it well. Savor the flavors.

Eating slowly is something you will have to do consciously at first. Your old habits will pop up from time to time and you'll probably catch yourself speeding up. You must resist your old habits to change them. Take smaller bites. Be aware of the contrasting colors, textures, and aromas. *Sip* (don't drink) a beverage with your meal, and be conscious of how its flavor intermingles with that of your food.

Another way to make eating a more satisfying experience is to make the atmosphere as attractive as possible. It's not an accident that fine restaurants usually have a lovely setting. The atmosphere enhances the food.

Set a proper table. Use your best china and silver. Never, never eat while standing up or on the run. If you do, you won't feel like you've eaten at all.

Don't do anything that will take your mind off the enjoyment of your food. For example, don't watch television. You are likely to become so involved in the action on the tube that you will forget about savoring your meal.

Soft music, candlelight, conversation, a deliberately relaxed pace, a beautiful table setting—all enhance the meal.

If mealtimes are particularly rushed at your house, find ways to slow them down. When you feel harried, you are more likely to eat too quickly and too much.

Allow yourself plenty of time for meal preparation. Snowbird recipes are all quick and simple, but try not to get into a frantic pace. If you are relaxed before the meal, you are more likely to be relaxed during the meal. Relaxation aids proper digestion of the food.

All Snowbird Recipes Have Been Professionally Tested

I have used some of these recipes for years—not just because they are low in calories, but because they are delicious. Still, compiling them into a book required precision and testing.

Kathleen Martin, a professional tester for *Bon Appétit* magazine, tested these recipes meticulously. Her expertise and care assure that each recipe will work in your kitchen exactly as it is intended. The recipes are precise and exact. However, if you would like to adjust the seasonings to suit your palate, that's perfectly fine.

The Recipes Are Quick and Simple

You don't want to spend hours in the kitchen when you are dieting (or even when you're not). Most of us lead busy lives today, so usually food preparation needs to be foolproof and fast.

Quick preparation is a cornerstone of Snowbird cuisine. And cleanup, the most dreaded of all kitchen chores, is a breeze because many of these dishes are prepared in throw-away foil packets.

THE SNOWBIRD KITCHEN

In the next few pages, I'll discuss some of the items that are indispensable to the Snowbird kitchen. These are the foods and seasonings that will make your kitchen a place where lifetime slenderness can thrive.

The Snowbird Pantry

Herbs

Cooking with herbs is a fine way to embellish the natural flavor of good food. Yet herbs are a mystery to many people.

Perla Myers, the noted cookbook author, explains herbs in a very simple way. She calls subtle ones "accent" herbs: chervil, parsley, chives, and dill. These are added at the end of cooking and give subtle accent to a dish.

Then there are "character" herbs: tarragon, rosemary, sweet basil, sage, oregano, marjoram, and thyme. These have a dominant flavor and are usually added to a dish while cooking. They add character to many dishes and are essential in ethnic cooking.

Snowbird Diet recipes use several various herbs to heighten flavor. Thanks to a growing demand, you are likely to find bunches of these fresh, aromatic sprigs in the produce section of your local market.

Growing your own herbs is easier today than ever, thanks to Frieda's Finest of California, which offers an assortment of potted herbs packaged for the supermarket (mint, chives, sweet basil, sage, rosemary, and thyme). They have serving suggestions on their twist ties and are widely available across the country. Your local nursery is also likely to have potted herbs ready for your windowsill or garden.

Fresh herbs can enhance the appearance of food as well as its flavor. For example, instead of garnishing a plate with the obligatory sprig of parsley, try using a fresh herb sprig such as tarragon, chervil, basil, or dill. It can add both flair and fragrance.

If you buy dried herbs, remember that their shelf life is not indefinite. As their green color pales, so does their flavor. Store dried herbs away from heat and light to prolong their goodness. Dried herbs are equal in flavor to twice the amount of fresh herbs.

In the following recipes, dried herbs are used, unless otherwise specified. However, if you are fortunate enough to have fresh herbs, just double the quantity called for.

Spices

While herbs consist of green plant leaves, spices are made from seeds or roots. They are available either ground or whole.

Curry powder is a good example of spice. It is actually a blend of many different ground spices.

Most seeds are too high in fat to be included in the Snowbird Diet, but one that we use often is nutmeg. You have probably used ground nutmeg, but for a real flavor treat, try whole nutmeg and grind it fresh. Whole nutmeg is available in many natural-food stores and kitchen-specialty shops. You will also need to get a nutmeg grater—a handy gadget that usually has a place to store nutmeg in the top, with a regular grater on the bottom. Tiny hand graters are also available. They, too, are generally available at cookware or food-specialty stores. Freshly grated nutmeg has a flavor completely different from the kind that comes preground. It is more pungent and the flavor almost sparkles. Use it to spark fresh fruits, yoghurt, spinach dishes, beef, chicken, and even chicken soup.

We also recommend allspice. It adds dimension to the flavors of vegetables and tomato dishes.

When flavoring foods with spices, use a light touch. The idea is to highlight the flavor, not to mask it.

Ginger is an extremely flavorful root that deserves some explanation. It is invaluable to delicious low-calorie cooking.

Ginger is available in many forms—candied, powdered, and pickled. We recommend fresh, whole ginger root for cooking. Powdered ginger is not an acceptable substitute for fresh.

Ginger root can usually be found in the produce section of your supermarket. It should look smooth, shiny, and plump. If it's wrinkled or dry-looking, it's past its prime.

Fresh ginger may be peeled, covered with dry sherry, and stored in a sealed container in your refrigerator. This way it will keep indefinitely. A nice bonus is the sherry, which develops a wonderful flavor and can be used for cooking and marinades.

Pepper

To get the most flavor from pepper, I suggest fresh, whole peppercorns and a good, small pepper mill.

Pepper loses much of its flavor and aroma after it has been ground, so using freshly ground pepper will really spark the flavor of your food.

There are many kinds of peppercorns: black (the most common); white (usually used on white foods such as potatoes, fish, rice, et cetera); cayenne (very hot—a little says a lot); green (these are found pickled whole and are used in the same manner as capers); and pink (expensive imports with delightful color and flavor). Crushed red peppers also add plenty of zing without adding calories.

Like other spices, peppercorns must be stored in a cool, dark place.

Mustard

A new wave of interest in mustards has grown so rapidly that there are now whole books devoted to this tangy condiment.

For the dieter, the boom in mustards is a windfall because mustard adds lots of pizzazz without adding any fat.

There is an abundance of new mustards available in most supermarkets today. Some are simple, some are exotic. There are domestics and imports. My favorite American version is made by Silver Palate.

The only mustards to avoid are those that are sweetened with honey, sugar, corn syrup, or any other form of sucrose. Check the labels before you buy.*

At a mere 5 calories per teaspoon, mustard offers many possibilities. Use it as a condiment, glaze, or basting ingredient for meats and poultry. Use it to flavor sauces for vegetables. When mixed with a bit of good vinegar, it makes a sensational salad dressing. Or, add mustard to commercial no-oil dressing for a tangy treat.

Try several different types of mustard. Mix and match them to produce new flavors. For example, start with Dijon and add your own flavorings—lemon zest (the yellow part of the rind only), crushed garlic, horseradish, ground pepper, or herbs.

Mustard travels well, too. It takes up almost no space and it doesn't need refrigeration.

Vinegar

It is well worth a trip to a gourmet food shop just to acquaint yourself with the vast array of delicious, fine-quality vinegars now available. You'll find vinegars made from red wine, white wine, blueberry,

*Other sugars to watch out for are mannitol, sorbitol, xylitol, maltase, and lactose, to name a few.

balsam, raspberry, apple cider, rice, champagne—the list goes on and on.

One of the best all-around vinegars I have found is sherry vinegar made by Silver Palate or La Posada (a Spanish import).

Vinegar makes an excellent marinade for meats and poultry. It can be used to deglaze a skillet for a lovely light sauce. Sprinkle it on fresh fruit or vegetable salads. And try it on poached fish.

If your vinegar tastes too sharp, dilute it with a bit of water. Always store vinegar in a cool, dark place.

Fats and Oils

Fats and oils are not unhealthful if they are eaten in small amounts. Since they are highly concentrated with calories, a tiny bit more than you should have can lead to unwanted pounds.

However, fats and oils in the proper portions are not only healthful and nutritionally important but add wonderful flavor.

Quality is extremely important here. Buy the very best you can.

When buying butter, select the unsalted type. Salt in butter acts as a preservative and may actually mask the flavor of rancid butter. Unsalted butter is fresher-tasting, and it lets you be the judge of how much salt goes into your food. Butter lasts longest when it is tightly wrapped and frozen.

There are as many kinds of oil on the market as there are vinegars. I recommend fine-quality olive oil. A 3-ounce bottle will last through this 12-day plan. If olive oil is not to your liking, peanut oil will suffice.

Chinese sesame oil (amber in color) and chili oil (to which crushed chili peppers have been added) are great seasoning oils. A few drops of either just before a dish is served can add lots of character.

It is best to buy oil in small quantity and store it in your refrigerator to keep it from going rancid.

Just one more point about oil: Many people are concerned about the difference between saturated and polyunsaturated fats in their diets. In the Snowbird Diet menus, so little oil is called for that it really makes little difference which kind you use.

Mushrooms

Mushrooms are a diet staple. They are low in fat and can be served in dozens of ways.

Today, many varieties are available in supermarkets and gourmet food shops. In addition to the ordinary button mushroom, there are dozens of imported dried varieties, from the Italian *porcini* to the Japanese *shiitake*. All add texture and flavor but very few calories.

Dried mushrooms must be reconstituted by soaking in hot water for at least 20 minutes. They should then be rinsed, drained, and prepared for use. The soaking liquid often takes on much flavor from the mushrooms and may be carefully strained and used in cooking. Dried mushrooms usually have a much stronger flavor than do fresh button mushrooms. For this reason, use less of them.

Fresh enoki mushrooms (long, skinny, and white) are now available in most supermarkets and are used in some of the following recipes.

When you bring home fresh mushrooms, don't wash them before they are refrigerated. Store them in a brown paper bag that is twisted shut. Before use, brush them clean or rinse briefly and dry immediately. Never let mushrooms soak in water or they will become waterlogged.

Select fresh mushrooms that are firm, white, and tightly closed. Once the cap has begun to open, the mushroom is past its prime.

Rice

More and more people are discovering what we have known for years—rice is healthful, versatile, and very important to the dieter.

Whether it is brown, wild,* or any of the many varieties of white rice now available, rice is amazingly nutritious and fat-free.

Because its natural flavor is delicate, rice can be combined with many different ingredients to make an endless array of dishes.

It's easy to cook rice from scratch. I recommend that you avoid precooked or quick-cooking rices. The regular types don't take that much longer to prepare and their flavors and textures are far superior.

To save cooking time later, cook a large batch of rice and freeze the extra in individual portions. Small servings defrost quickly for last-minute meals.

Experiment with different rices—pearl, short-, medium-, or long-grain—but avoid rice mixes.

---

*Technically, wild rice is an aquatic grass, not a rice.

Cooking with Wine

Wine adds lots of flavor to food, and almost all the calories evaporate with the alcohol during cooking.

When you cook with wine, sherry, or vermouth, always select a variety that is dry. The better quality you use, the better-tasting your dish will be. A good rule of thumb is that if it's not good to drink, it's not good for cooking.

The Snowbird Diet allows you to have a 4-ounce glass of wine each day, but if you decide to save those extra calories, you needn't buy a bottle of wine just for cooking. Use dry vermouth or sherry instead. They can be purchased in small bottles and will last indefinitely after they have been opened.

As you will discover in the following recipes, it is necessary to boil away the alcohol after it is added to a dish. Do this by bringing the dish to a boil and then simmering it for about 3 minutes. The calories and alcohol will both evaporate.

Flavor Wrap-Up

Many of the dishes on the Snowbird Diet are cooked in tightly wrapped packets of heavy-duty aluminum foil. This produces results similar to the French method of cooking *en papillote*, in which food is encased in buttered parchment paper. Using foil eliminates the calories that come with buttered paper, but it achieves the same result. Food cooks in its own juice, retaining its flavor and nutrients.

Wrap the food in a generous piece of foil so that it is completely enclosed, then seal it tightly to prevent moisture from escaping.

Cooking in foil packets makes both cooking and cleanup a snap, and, if you wish, you may bring individual packets right to the table, where they can be opened by each diner.

Leftovers are easy, too, because they may be refrigerated and reheated in the same foil wrap.

Beverages

In addition to your daily water requirement, you may also enjoy other low-calorie beverages. Remember that caffeinated drinks are to be avoided. And if you are salt-sensitive, limit your intake of diet soft drinks to those that are salt-, sugar-, and caffeine-free.

You are entitled to one cocktail per day. Select a 4-ounce glass of dry wine,* a light beer, or one shot (1½ ounces) of hard liquor mixed with a low-calorie mixer.† Here are some things to keep in mind should you exercise your cocktail option:

- The calories and carbohydrates in cocktails are **not** included in the daily totals. They are in addition to those counts.
- Any alcoholic beverage you consume will add calories† and therefore make weight loss slower.
- Alcoholic drinks may lower inhibitions and increase the appetite. It is best to have your drink with dinner rather than before. You may not be as tempted to overeat.

If you opt not to indulge in alcohol, here are some of the light, refreshing, nonalcoholic drinks we recommend:

- Perrier with a dash of bitters
- Virgin Mary
- Virgin Bull
- Low-Cal Cranapple Spritzer
- Scottsdale Spritz—2 ounces dry red wine with soda and a twist of lemon
- V-8 Juice and soda
- Low-Cal Cranberry Cocktail with low-cal tonic
- Arizona sun tea—4 bags of tea in a 2-quart clear glass jar filled with cold water. Put a lid on the jar and place outside in the sun for several hours. This makes delicious, strong tea that doesn't cloud. Refrigerate the bottle. Dilute with water to desired strength when serving. Pour over ice and garnish with a sprig of fresh mint. Arizona sun tea can be made almost anywhere, anytime the sun is out. One friend of ours made it in Minneapolis in March! In cold weather, double the number of tea bags and keep an eye on the container if the temperature dips below freezing.

*If you normally drink white wine, you might want to switch to red or rosé. These, more than white wine, increase your taste awareness.

†To estimate the calories in alcohol, use this formula: 1 calorie per proof per ounce.

Vitamin and Mineral Supplements

The Snowbird Diet is low in calories and fat and very high in nutrients. Even so, we recommend that patients supplement the diet with the following:

    1. One Miles Laboratory 1-A-Day Vitamins with Minerals and Iron. Do not consume coffee or tea within 1 hour of taking the supplement. Foods high in vitamin C (citrus fruits, broccoli, et cetera) will enhance the absorption from the supplement.

    2. Calcium: 1,000 mg. per day for men and premenopausal women; 1,500 mg. per day for postmenopausal women. Os-Cal is a good brand, easy to obtain; but there are many others that are suitable. Do not take calcium if you have had a problem with kidney stones unless you consult your physician. Calcium may be taken anytime, but most patients find that taking it at night helps induce sleep and aids absorption.

What If You Can't Eat This Much Food?

We have often heard, "I just can't eat this much food. What should I do?"

    If you find yourself asking that question, cut back on everything **except** the protein. It's fine to reduce the servings of fruits, vegetables, and complex carbohydrates, but you must eat *all* the protein that is recommended.

Additional Protein Recommended for Some

While the Snowbird Diet contains generous amounts of protein, all men whose ideal (goal) weight is 190 pounds or more need to add more protein. We recommend that these men add either 12 ounces buttermilk (made from skim or low-fat milk) **or** 12 ounces skim (nonfat) milk *per day*.

Snowbird Shopping

For your convenience, you will find detailed shopping lists for every three days of the diet after every three days' menus. They are complete.

Everything you will need for the diet is listed.

Buy only the freshest and finest ingredients available. The fresher and better the food, the tastier and more nutritious it will be.

Since you will be buying less food overall, you can afford better quality.

When produce looks wilted or past its prime, select good-quality frozen or canned products.

When Should You Start the Diet?

The Snowbird Diet is geared to start on Monday morning. That's when most people feel good about starting a weight-control program. We have designed menus for each day of the week, and on the weekend there are special brunches.

If you decide to start the diet on a day other than Monday, be sure to begin with Day 1 just the same. It will keep your shopping lists in order and the nutrition in a sequence that will promote quicker weight loss.

All Recipes Serve Two

All the Snowbird recipes make two servings, unless otherwise noted. To serve more or fewer than two people, simply adjust the recipes accordingly. If you are cooking for one, it's a real time saver to cook both portions and freeze one for later use. **Do not** eat more than the one serving of any of the foods. Remember, low-calorie meals are not low-calorie if you eat twice as much as you should.

About the Diet

The daily menus for the next 12 days are simple and self-explanatory. If you have a question, the answer can probably be found in chapter 12, "Snowbird Dieters Ask the Doctor."

If there are foods on the menu that you can't eat, refer to the Emergency Food Plan for alternatives. Read the instructions for using the Emergency Food Plan carefully *before* you make any substitutions.

DAY 1—MONDAY

Breakfast

Sliced Kiwi Fruit

Soft-Boiled Egg

Kavli (Norwegian Crisp Flat Bread)

Lunch

Seafood Salad

Dinner

Ginger Chicken

Rice

Steamed Fresh Chinese Pea Pods

Swiss Chard and Bibb Lettuce Salad

Paradise Valley Parfait

Breakfast

Preparation time: 10 minutes

2 kiwis, peeled and sliced (1 per person, 7 ounces total)
2 soft-boiled eggs (1 per person)

4 pieces Kavli (2 whole wafers per person)

	CAL	CHO	PR	F&O*†
Recipe Totals	408	59	16	11
Serving Totals	204	30	8	6

Lunch

SEAFOOD SALAD

Preparation time: 30 minutes

This dish must be prepared in advance so that the gelatin can set. Make it in the morning, or even one day ahead.

2 cups spicy V-8 Juice
1 envelope unflavored gelatin
1 teaspoon dried sweet basil
1 7-ounce can lobster or water-pack tuna, drained
3 tablespoons diced green bell pepper

3 tablespoons radish slices (2 medium)
2 tablespoons scallion slices (1 large)
Garnish: 4 red lettuce leaves

Measure 1 cup V-8 Juice into pan. Sprinkle juice with gelatin. Let gelatin soften for 5 minutes. Add basil. Heat mixture over medium

*Calories (CAL), Complex Carbohydrates (CHO), Protein (PR), and Fats and Oils (F&O)

†When totals for recipes were odd numbers, serving totals have been rounded up to the next higher number.

heat until gelatin is dissolved and juice is steamy but not boiling. Add remaining cup of V-8 Juice. Chill 1 hour. Fold in remaining ingredients. Chill until set. Serve each portion on 2 red lettuce leaves.

	CAL	CHO	PR	F&O
Recipe Totals	339	29	45	3
Serving Totals	170	15	23	2

Dinner

GINGER CHICKEN

Preparation time: 30 minutes

Fresh ginger is potent, so use it judiciously

2 7-ounce chicken breasts, skinned and boned
⅛ teaspoon pepper
1 ounce fresh ginger root, peeled and minced
4 water chestnuts, sliced
4 scallions
1 tablespoon soy sauce
1 cup cooked rice*
2 teaspoons parsley, chopped

Place each piece of chicken in its own piece of heavy-duty aluminum foil. Sprinkle each with pepper, ginger, and sliced water chestnuts. Top each with 2 whole scallions. Divide soy sauce between each packet, sprinkling evenly over all. Seal tightly and steam 25 minutes in oven at 350°, or in steamer. To serve, open packet and pour juices over cooked rice. Arrange chicken on the side and garnish with chopped parsley. Store leftover water chestnuts covered with water in the refrigerator. Change water daily.

*To save time, consider cooking twice as much rice as you need tonight and save the rest for lunch tomorrow.

GINGER CHICKEN	CAL	CHO	PR	F&O
Recipe Totals—Chicken	490	19	83	5
Serving Totals	245	10	42	3
Recipe Totals—Rice	164	36	3	0
Serving Totals	82	18	2	0

STEAMED FRESH CHINESE PEA PODS

Preparation time: 10 minutes

1 cup fresh Chinese pea pods

Remove strings from pea pods. Steam 3 to 5 minutes until tender-crisp.

	CAL	CHO	PR	F&O
Recipe Totals	43	9	3	0
Serving Totals	22	5	2	0

SWISS CHARD SALAD

Preparation time: 5 minutes

2 cups Swiss chard, washed and dried
2 tablespoons sherry vinegar
1 teaspoon Dijon mustard
2 cups torn Bibb lettuce

Remove stems from Swiss chard and tear into bite-size pieces. Combine sherry vinegar and mustard, mix until smooth. Pour dressing over lettuce and toss lightly. Serve immediately. Salt and pepper at table as desired.

	CAL	CHO	PR	F&O
Recipe Totals	62	11	5	0
Serving Totals	31	6	3	0

PARADISE VALLEY PARFAIT

Preparation time: 10 minutes

1½ cups cubed fresh,
    ripe pineapple
½ cup plain low-fat yoghurt

Sprinkling of ground nutmeg

Mix pineapple with yoghurt. Sprinkle with nutmeg.

	CAL	CHO	PR	F&O
Recipe Totals	160	31	7	1
Serving Totals	80	16	4	1
Daily Totals	1666	194	162	20
Totals Per Person	833	97	81	10

DAY 2—TUESDAY

Breakfast

Banana Blend

Lunch

Crabmeat Salad with Rice

Dinner

Caviar Consommé

Steak Tartare

Asparagus Spears on Lettuce

Lahvosh (Armenian Cracker Bread)

Pear Baked in Red Wine

Breakfast

BANANA BLEND

Preparation time: 5 minutes

½ cup water
½ cup nonfat dry milk
1 banana (6 ounces)

⅛ teaspoon ground cinnamon
4 ice cubes

Combine first four ingredients. Blend for 30 seconds. Add ice cubes and blend an additional 15 seconds, or until smooth. Makes two 1-cup servings. Add more water if too thick for your taste.

	CAL	CHO	PR	F&O
Recipe Totals	192	38	11	0
Serving Totals	96	19	6	0

Lunch

CRABMEAT SALAD WITH RICE

Preparation time: 10 minutes

This is especially easy if you use leftover rice from last night's dinner. It can be made early in the morning if your lunchtime is rushed.

1 6½-ounce can crabmeat
 (or fresh if available)
1 cup cooked rice
3 tablespoons any no-oil
 dressing
¼ cup finely chopped celery

2 whole scallions, chopped
 (4 tablespoons)
⅛ teaspoon pepper
½ teaspoon curry powder
1 teaspoon lemon juice
3½ ounces lettuce (any type)

Combine all ingredients except lettuce and mix well. Arrange each serving on half the lettuce.

	CAL	CHO	PR	F&O
Recipe Totals	410	48	39	4
Serving Totals	205	24	20	2

Dinner

CAVIAR CONSOMMÉ

Preparation time: 5 minutes

This soup may also be served hot.

1 13-ounce can consommé, well-chilled (Crosse and Blackwell Red Consommé Madrilene is best)
2 tablespoons plain low-fat yoghurt
4 teaspoons caviar (any from lumpfish to beluga)
1 scant teaspoon finely grated lemon zest (yellow part of the lemon rind only)

Divide cold consommé in half. Top each serving with half the yoghurt. Top with half the caviar and a sprinkling of lemon zest.

	CAL	CHO	PR	F&O
Recipe Totals	164	11	14	7
Serving Totals	82	6	7	4

STEAK TARTARE

Preparation time: 20 minutes

Packaged ground meat is unacceptable for this dish. You must buy fresh top-round steak. Have your butcher trim away *all* visible fat and grind it, or you can grind it in a food processor or grinder.

For those who do not eat raw beef, steak tartare may be broiled.

An attractive way to serve this dish is to arrange lettuce leaves on a serving plate. Place the steak tartare on the lettuce and surround with asparagus spears. Garnish with capers and thinly sliced red onion.

Capers are a flavorful addition to many foods, and they add very few calories. They are the pickled bud of a bush that grows wild in Europe and Asia.

6 ounces freshly ground top round steak (no packaged meat)
1 egg yolk, slightly beaten
½ onion, finely chopped
2 tablespoons parsley

1 tablespoon capers
½ teaspoon salt
⅛ teaspoon pepper
⅛ teaspoon minced garlic
3 drops Tabasco sauce

Mix egg with ground round. Work in remaining ingredients. Form into two patties.

	CAL	CHO	PR	F&O
Recipe Totals	524	6	59	28
Serving Totals	262	3	30	14

ASPARAGUS SPEARS ON LETTUCE

Preparation time: 10 minutes

12 asparagus spears (fresh or frozen), steamed 6 minutes or to desired degree of tenderness, with ½ teaspoon salt and ¼ teaspoon pepper

1 tablespoon no-oil dressing
1 teaspoon sherry vinegar
⅛ teaspoon crushed garlic
4 large lettuce leaves (any type)
4 thin slices of red onion

To the no-oil dressing add sherry vinegar and crushed garlic. Sprinkle over warm asparagus. Marinate no longer than 1 hour. Arrange asparagus around steak tartare on lettuce leaves. Garnish with sliced onion.

	CAL	CHO	PR	F&O
Recipe Totals	80	13	9	0
Serving Totals	40	7	5	0

PEAR BAKED IN RED WINE

Preparation time: 10 minutes

You may use any type of pear for this recipe. (Since you are poaching the pear, it is not necessary for the pear to be *very* ripe.) Use the best dry red wine possible. You may use a low-calorie sweetener, but it is best to allow the natural sugar in the pear to shine through.

1 pear, sliced lengthwise and cored

½ cup dry red wine

Bring wine to a boil and simmer uncovered for 3 minutes to allow the alcohol to evaporate. Add pear halves, cover, and simmer 5 to 8 minutes. Serve warm or cold.

	CAL	CHO	PR	F&O
Recipe Totals	138	35	1	1
Serving Totals	69	18	1	1

LAHVOSH (Armenian Cracker Bread)

1 5-inch cracker per person

	CAL	CHO	PR	F&O
Recipe totals	117	19	5	2
Serving Totals	59	10	3	1
Daily Totals	1625	170	138	42
Totals Per Person	813	85	69	21

DAY 3—WEDNESDAY

Breakfast
Tomato and Chèvre on Flatbread
Lunch
Grande Gazpacho
Blackened Beef Tartare
Marinated Mushroom Salad
Dinner
Italian Shrimp
Rice
Patio Salad
Grilled Fresh Pineapple

Breakfast

TOMATO AND CHÈVRE ON FLATBREAD

Preparation time: 10 minutes

Chèvre, or goat cheese, is flavorful and low in fat. Many varieties are now available, both domestic and imported. If you cannot find chèvre, use feta. If the feta tastes too salty, soak it in cold water for a few minutes to release the salt. Pat dry before serving.

1 large tomato, sliced thin and divided	¼ teaspoon crushed sweet basil (optional)
1½ ounces chèvre or 2 ounces feta	⅛ teaspoon pepper (optional)
4 Kavli wafers	

Divide tomato and cheese among four Kavli wafers. Can be served cold or warmed under the broiler.

	CAL	CHO	PR	F&O
Recipe Totals	321	39	14	12
Serving Totals	161	20	7	6

Lunch

GRANDE GAZPACHO

Preparation time: 25 minutes

For convenience, this soup may be made a day ahead and chilled overnight.

1 12-ounce can V-8 Juice
1 tomato, cored and chopped (¾ cup)
2 scallions, chopped (4 tablespoons)
¼ green bell pepper, diced

3 drops Tabasco sauce
½ teaspoon salt
⅛ teaspoon pepper
1½ teaspoons minced parsley
¼ teaspoon thyme
¼ teaspoon sweet basil

Combine all ingredients. Season to taste and chill thoroughly (3–4 hours or overnight).

	CAL	CHO	PR	F&O
Recipe Totals	109	24	5	0
Serving Totals	55	12	3	0

BLACKENED BEEF TARTARE

Preparation time: 15 minutes

10 ounces freshly chopped ground round
3 drops Tabasco sauce
1 tablespoon minced parsley
2 tablespoons minced scallions

½ teaspoon thyme
½ teaspoon salt
⅛ teaspoon pepper
1 tablespoon Dijon mustard
Garnish: lemon wedges

Combine all ingredients. Make two 5-ounce patties. Fry in nonstick pan without oil. Drain on paper towels. Garnish with lemon wedge.

BLACKENED BEEF TARTARE	CAL	CHO	PR	F&O
Recipe Totals	554	6	58	32
Serving Totals	277	3	29	16

MARINATED MUSHROOM SALAD

Preparation time: 10 minutes

16 large mushrooms, sliced
   (12 ounces)
½ teaspoon salt
⅛ teaspoon pepper
 1 teaspoon lemon juice
 1 tablespoon minced parsley

½ teaspoon sweet basil
 2 tablespoons no-oil
   dressing mixed with 2
   tablespoons sherry vinegar
3½ ounces lettuce (any type)

Sprinkle mushrooms with salt, pepper, and lemon juice. Toss lightly. Add parsley, basil, and dressing. Toss again. Marinate, covered with plastic wrap, for 1 hour. Serve over lettuce.

	CAL	CHO	PR	F&O
Recipe Totals	77	11	7	0
Serving Totals	39	6	4	0

Dinner

ITALIAN SHRIMP

Preparation time: 30 minutes

12 ounces peeled, deveined shrimp (fresh or frozen)
5½ ounces zucchini, sliced (1 medium)
1 8-ounce tomato, coarsely chopped (¾ cup)
2 scallions, chopped (4 tablespoons)

¾ teaspoon salt
1 teaspoon sweet basil
1 teaspoon minced garlic
¼ teaspoon pepper
2 tablespoons no-oil dressing
1 cup hot cooked rice

Divide first 8 ingredients in half and arrange on individual pieces of heavy-duty aluminum foil. Drizzle each with 1 tablespoon of the dressing. Seal tightly and steam for 10 minutes. Open packets and pour juices over ½ cup rice. Arrange shrimp on the side.

	CAL	CHO	PR	F&O
Recipe Totals—Shrimp	391	22	64	3
Serving Totals	196	11	32	2
Recipe Totals—Rice	164	36	3	0
Serving Totals	82	18	2	0

PATIO SALAD

Preparation time: 5–10 minutes

2 cups romaine lettuce
1 cup chicory
1 cup lettuce of your choice
  (depending upon which
  looks freshest and best at
  the market)

2 tablespoons no-oil dressing
  Salt and freshly ground
  pepper

Wash and dry greens. Tear into bite-size pieces. Toss lightly with dressing. Add salt and pepper to taste.

	CAL	CHO	PR	F&O
Recipe Totals	41	8	1	0
Serving Totals	21	4	1	0

GRILLED FRESH PINEAPPLE

Preparation time: 5 minutes

2 slices fresh pineapple, ¾
  inch thick and 3½ inches
  long.

Grill pineapple (or broil) until lightly browned. Serve warm.

	CAL	CHO	PR	F&O
Recipe Totals	88	23	1	0
Serving Totals	44	12	1	0
Daily Totals	1745	169	153	47
Totals Per Person	873	85	77	24

SHOPPING LIST
DAYS 1, 2, 3

shrimp (12 oz.)
boneless chicken breasts (2)
   (7 oz. each)
top round steak, ground (1 lb.)
eggs (1 doz.)
plain low-fat yoghurt
   (1 container) (8 oz.)
feta cheese (11 oz.)
capers (3¼ oz.)
kiwis (2)
banana (1)
lemons (2)
pear (1)
pineapple (1)
Chinese pea pods (1 cup)
fresh Swiss chard
   (2 cups leaves)
Bibb lettuce (2 cups)
green pepper (1)
scallions (10)
red lettuce (1 head)
ginger root (1)
asparagus spears (16)
red onion (1)
celery (1 small bunch)
onions (2)
tomatoes (3)
mushrooms (16) (or 12 oz.)
zucchini (1 medium)
radishes (1 bunch)
romaine (1 head)
chicory (1 head)

parsley (1 bunch)
Kavli Norwegian flatbread (1
   pkg.) (5¾ oz.)
whole-grain white rice (1 box)
   (11½ cups)
powdered skim milk (9.6 oz.)
low-calorie sweetener
unflavored gelatin (1 packet)
Lahvosh
heavy-duty foil
no-oil dressing (12 oz.)
Tabasco (2 oz.)
sherry vinegar (1 bottle)
soy sauce
lobster or albacore tuna (1 can)
   (7 oz.)
V-8 Juice (1 can) (12 oz.)
V-8 (hot and spicy) (three 6-oz.
   cans or one 12-oz. and one 6-
   oz. can)
crabmeat (6½ oz.)
consommé—well chilled (1 can)
   (Crosse and Blackwell Red
   Consommé Madrilene)
caviar (2 oz.)
water chestnuts (1 small can)
basil
thyme
garlic head (1)
cinnamon
curry powder
nutmeg

DAY 4—THURSDAY

Breakfast
Canadian Bacon
Baguette
Hot Virgin Bloody Bull
Lunch
Chicken Broth with Escarole
Smoked Salmon Omelette
Dinner
Cornish Game Hen Dijonnaise
Green Beans
Puffed New Potato
Surprise Salad
Raspberries

Breakfast

CANADIAN BACON

Preparation time: 5 minutes

8 slices Canadian bacon,
⅛ inch thick (4 ounces)

Heat a nonstick skillet for 2 minutes over medium heat. Sauté Canadian bacon for two minutes on one side. Turn bacon over and sauté an additional 30 seconds. The meat will be lightly browned and moist.

	CAL	CHO	PR	F&O
Recipe Totals	156	1	24	7
Serving Totals	78	1	12	4

BAGUETTE

4 thin slices baguette
(2 ounces)

	CAL	CHO	PR	F&O
Recipe Totals	174	34	6	2
Serving Totals	87	17	3	1

HOT VIRGIN BLOODY BULL

Preparation time: 5 minutes

1 can tomato juice
(12 ounces)
1 can beef consommé, full
strength (10½ ounces)

½ teaspoon Angostura Bitters
2 lemon wedges

Combine juice and consommé. Heat over medium heat for 3–4 minutes. Add bitters. Serve with lemon wedge.

	CAL	CHO	PR	F&O
Recipe Totals	104	16	3	0
Serving Totals	52	8	2	0

Lunch

CHICKEN BROTH WITH ESCAROLE

Preparation time: 10 minutes

Be sure to trim enoki mushrooms down at least 1 inch from root base.

1   can chicken broth (14½ ounces)
1½ ounces dry white wine
½ cup enoki mushrooms (1 ounce)

2 cups escarole leaves or curly endive (2 ounces)
⅛ teaspoon pepper

Refrigerate broth overnight so that congealed fat will stick to the lid when the can is opened. Remove any remaining fat with a spoon. Place broth and wine into a pan. Heat over medium heat for 5 minutes until broth simmers. Meanwhile, clean escarole leaves and chop into 1-inch pieces. Add mushrooms and escarole to broth. Simmer uncovered for 10 minutes. Serve hot.

	CAL	CHO	PR	F&O
Recipe Totals	123	16	9	4
Serving Totals	62	8	5	2

SMOKED SALMON OMELETTE

Preparation time: 35 minutes

Today's lunch travels well if you're thinking of a picnic or even work. The omelette should be served at room temperature, and the soup will stay piping hot in a thermos.

2 whole eggs
2 egg whites
Pinch of cream of tartar
⅛ teaspoon salt
Pinch of pepper

2 ounces feta or 1½ ounces chèvre
3½ ounces smoked salmon
½ cup packed watercress, leaves and tender shoots only

Put whole eggs and whites together in a bowl with cream of tartar. Heat a nonstick skillet for 2 minutes over medium heat. Beat eggs with a whisk until light and frothy. Pour into pan, reduce heat as low as possible, cover, and let rest three minutes or until eggs are set. Season with salt and pepper. Crumble cheese over surface, cover with salmon and watercress.

Gently slide omelette onto a piece of plastic wrap. Using plastic wrap to help lift the eggs, roll the omelette as tight as possible, twist the ends, and tuck the ends under the roll. Chill. Remove from refrigerator, slice into 1-inch slices, and garnish with additional watercress. May be prepared one day in advance.

	CAL	CHO	PR	F&O
Recipe Totals	509	4	53	31
Serving Totals	255	2	27	16

Dinner

CORNISH GAME HENS DIJONNAISE

Preparation time: 1 hour 15 minutes

2 Cornish game hens
(22 ounces each)
¼ cup Dijon mustard
2 tablespoons fresh grapefruit
juice

⅛ teaspoon cracked pepper
2 teaspoons grapefruit zest
(yellow of rind only)

Combine mustard, grapefruit juice, pepper, and zest. Using your fingers, carefully separate the skin from the flesh of the hens. Spread mustard mixture between skin and flesh, covering meaty parts well. Roast on a rack at 350° for 45 minutes. Raise temperature to 400°. Add potatoes (see page 90). Continue baking for an additional 15 minutes. Remove hens from oven and let rest, covered loosely with foil, for 15 minutes while potatoes finish baking. Cut hens in half. Reserve one hen for tomorrow's lunch. Remove skin from tonight's portions and discard. Sprinkle liberally with cracked pepper and serve.

	CAL	CHO	PR	F&O
Recipe Totals	231	2	37	7
Serving Totals	116	1	19	4

GREEN BEANS

Preparation time: 20 minutes

2 cups fresh green beans   ¾ teaspoon thyme
  (11 ounces)

Trim ends of beans and snap into 1-inch pieces. After trimming there will be nine ounces of beans. Put ½ inch of water and the thyme in a pot. Bring water to a boil. Add beans to a steamer basket that fits into the pot. Cover and steam for 13 minutes.

	CAL	CHO	PR	F&O
Recipe Totals	62	14	4	0
Serving Totals	31	7	2	0

PUFFED RED POTATOES

Preparation time: 35 minutes

2 small red potatoes   ⅛ teaspoon salt
  (3½ ounces each)

Cut washed potatoes in half. Sprinkle with salt and place in oven cut side up when you raise the temperature to 400° for the game hens. Bake a total of 30 minutes. Potatoes will puff and brown. Season with pepper if desired.

	CAL	CHO	PR	F&O
Recipe Totals	152	34	4	0
Serving Totals	76	17	2	0

SURPRISE SALAD

Preparation time: 10 minutes

1¼ cups shredded red
   cabbage
½ small apple (3-inch
   diameter), cored and diced
1 tablespoon fresh
   grapefruit juice

2 tablespoons plain
   low-fat yoghurt
¼ teaspoon caraway seeds
   or poppy seeds
⅛ teaspoon salt

Place cabbage in a bowl. Toss apple and grapefruit juice and add to cabbage. Combine yoghurt, seeds, and salt. Add to cabbage mixture and toss to coat. Cover with plastic wrap and marinate in the refrigerator for 1 hour.

	CAL	CHO	PR	F&O
Recipe Totals	103	22	4	1
Serving Totals	52	11	2	1

RASPBERRIES

Preparation time: 1 minute

1½ cups fresh or unsweetened
frozen raspberries

Rinse fruit and serve.

	CAL	CHO	PR	F&O
Recipe Totals	114	27	2	0
Serving Totals	57	14	1	0
Daily Totals	1728	170	146	52
Totals Per Person	864	85	73	26

DAY 5—FRIDAY

Breakfast

Sliced Kiwi Fruit

Soft-Boiled Egg

Kavli

Lunch

Cold Cornish Game Hen

Hot Curried Yoghurt Soup

Dinner

Lobster Tail with Endive and Fennel

Spinach Salad with Enoki Mushrooms

Baguette

Banana Sidney

Breakfast

Same as Day 1

Lunch

COLD CORNISH GAME HEN

Preparation time: 5 minutes

1 Cornish game hen left from
last night (½ per person)

Skin the hen just before lunch to retain flavor and moisture. Discard
skin. Sprinkle hen with cracked pepper if desired.

	CAL	CHO	PR	F&O
Recipe Totals	231	2	37	7
Serving Totals	116	1	19	4

HOT CURRIED YOGHURT SOUP

Preparation time: 10 minutes

This soup is wonderful either hot or cold. If you are not accustomed
to curry, you may want to add a bit less at first.

1 can chicken broth
(14½ ounces—canned or
homemade)
1 cup cucumber, halved,
seeded, and sliced ⅛ inch
thick

1 cup plain low-fat yoghurt
1 teaspoon curry powder
Pinch of cayenne pepper

Refrigerate broth so that congealed fat can be removed easily. Remove fat and heat broth over medium heat for 5 minutes until simmering. Add cucumber slices and simmer 4 minutes. Reduce heat as low as possible. Mix yoghurt, curry, and cayenne pepper. Whisk into soup. Do not boil or soup will curdle.

	CAL	CHO	PR	F&O
Recipe Totals	223	24	16	7
Serving Totals	112	12	8	4

Dinner

LOBSTER TAILS WITH ENDIVE AND FENNEL*

Preparation time: 30 minutes

3½ cups fennel (sweet anise), root and stalks (10 ounces)

2 cups Belgian endive (7 ounces)

½ teaspoon olive oil lobster tail, fresh or defrosted in shell (14 ounces)

2 teaspoons lemon juice

½ teaspoon salt

⅛ teaspoon freshly ground pepper

½ cup white wine

⅛ to ¼ teaspoon paprika

Remove tough ends of fennel root and slice into ½-inch slices. Using a vegetable peeler, peel fennel stalks to remove tough exterior and slice into ½-inch pieces. Cut endive in half, lengthwise, and remove core. Heat a nonstick skillet for 2 minutes over medium heat. Put olive oil in skillet. Shake the skillet to distribute the oil over the surface. Add fennel, toss with oil, cover, and cook 5 minutes.

Slit lobster down length of tail with a sharp knife, cutting through

*Celery or jicama may be substituted for fennel with only a slight variation in nutrient composition of recipe.

only the belly side of the shell (not the back of the lobster), so that the tail will retain its shape in one piece. Sprinkle with 1 teaspoon lemon juice and a scant ¼ teaspoon salt. Add endive and another scant ¼ teaspoon salt plus the pepper and wine to the skillet. Mix to combine flavors.

Place lobster on top of vegetables, cover, and steam 10 minutes. Remove lobster and set aside. With a slotted spoon, arrange the vegetables on two ovenproof plates. Place in a 300° oven.

Turn heat under skillet to high. Add remaining 1 teaspoon of lemon juice. Reduce liquid until you have about 2 tablespoons. Spoon 1 tablespoon of the juice over each serving. Sprinkle with paprika and serve at once.

LOBSTER TAILS WITH ENDIVE AND FENNEL	CAL	CHO	PR	F&O
Recipe Totals	345	28	47	6
Serving Totals	173	14	24	3

SPINACH SALAD WITH ENOKI MUSHROOMS

Preparation time: 20 minutes

1 **bunch fresh spinach
(5 ounces or 2 cups
packed raw)**
½ **cup enoki mushrooms
(1 ounce)**
3 **tablespoons no-oil dressing**

2 **teaspoons sherry vinegar
Scant ½ teaspoon salt**
⅛ **teaspoon pepper**
⅛ **teaspoon minced garlic**

Wash and dry spinach. Remove stems and tear leaves into bite-size pieces. Cut tough root end off mushrooms. In a small bowl, mix no-oil dressing, vinegar, salt, pepper, and garlic. Toss spinach and mushrooms with dressing.

	CAL	CHO	PR	F&O
Recipe Totals	83	13	7	0
Serving Totals	42	7	4	0

BAGUETTE

Same as Breakfast, Day 4 (4
thin slices or 2 ounces)

BANANA SIDNEY

Preparation time: 5 minutes

1 6-ounce banana, peeled and
sliced lengthwise
3 tablespoons plain low-fat
yoghurt

1 packet low-calorie sweetener
(1 gram)
Freshly grated nutmeg or
cinnamon

Heat a nonstick skillet over medium heat for 1 minute. Place banana,
cut side down, in skillet and cook 1 minute. Mix yoghurt and sweetener.
Put the banana halves on separate plates. Top each with half the
yoghurt and sprinkle with nutmeg or cinnamon.

	CAL	CHO	PR	F&O
Recipe Totals	142	35	3	0
Serving Totals	71	18	2	0
Daily Totals	1606	195	132	33
Totals Per Person	803	98	66	17

DAY 6—SATURDAY

Brunch

Raspberries in Champagne

Chèvre and Spinach Omelette

Wheat Lahvosh with Tomato

Dinner

Veal Chops with Salsa of Peppers

Steamed New Potatoes

Hearts of Palm Salad

Broiled Orange

Brunch

RASPBERRIES IN CHAMPAGNE

Preparation time: 2 minutes

(Obviously, you will lose more weight if you do not have alcoholic beverages. But if you choose to drink champagne it must count as your daily allowance of alcohol. If champagne is not to your liking, eliminate it or substitute with low-calorie ginger ale.)

1½ cups raspberries (fresh or partially frozen, unsweetened)

1 cup cold champagne or low-calorie ginger ale
Fresh mint sprigs (optional)

Divide the raspberries between two large goblets. Pour champagne over berries. Garnish with mint.

	CAL	CHO	PR	F&O
Recipe Totals	282	33	2	0
Serving Totals	141	17	1	0

CHÈVRE AND SPINACH OMELETTE

Preparation time: 20 minutes

2 whole eggs
2 egg whites
Pinch of cream of tartar
1 cup fresh spinach leaves, finely chopped

⅛ teaspoon salt
Pinch of pepper
1½ ounces chèvre or 2 ounces feta

In a mixing bowl, beat eggs and egg whites with cream of tartar. Heat a nonstick skillet for 2 minutes over medium heat. Beat eggs with a whisk until light and frothy. Add spinach. Pour into pan, reduce heat as low as possible, cover, and let rest 4 minutes or until eggs are set. Season with salt and pepper.

Loosen omelette from sides and bottom of skillet with spatula. Crumble cheese over half the omelette. Fold the other half of the omelette over the cheese. Let rest 1 minute, uncovered, then divide in half and serve.

	CAL	CHO	PR	F&O
Recipe Totals	356	7	34	22
Serving Totals	178	4	17	11

WHEAT LAHVOSH WITH TOMATO

Preparation time: 5 minutes

2 5-inch wheat Lahvosh
1 medium tomato cut into 6 slices
⅛ teaspoon salt

Pinch of pepper
¼ teaspoon sweet basil
1 teaspoon minced chives

Arrange 3 tomato slices on each Lahvosh. Season with salt, pepper, basil, and chives.

	CAL	CHO	PR	F&O
Recipe Totals	139	24	6	2
Serving Totals	70	12	3	1

Dinner

VEAL CHOPS WITH SALSA OF PEPPERS

Preparation time: 25 minutes

2 veal chops ¾-inch thick trimmed of all visible fat (1 pound raw with bone)
¼ teaspoon salt
Pinch of pepper
1 teaspoon olive oil
3½ ounces dry wine

½ teaspoon sweet basil minced together with
1 tablespoon parsley and
1 clove garlic
1¼ cups each red and green bell pepper, seeded and sliced ½-inch thick

Heat a nonstick skillet over medium heat for 1 minute. Season chops with salt and pepper. Add olive oil to skillet and shake pan to distribute oil over surface. Add chops and sauté 2 minutes on each side. Turn heat to medium low, cover, and cook 3 minutes. Turn chops over, cover, and cook an additional 3 minutes.

Remove chops from skillet, place on warm plate, and keep warm, covered loosely with foil, in a 140° oven. Pour wine into skillet and turn heat to high, stirring to combine all brown bits. Add basil mixture and peppers and toss to coat. Reduce heat to medium, cover, and cook 5 minutes. Pour any juices from veal into skillet. Remove peppers and arrange them around veal. Pour pan juices over.

	CAL	CHO	PR	F&O
Recipe Totals	741	16	93	32
Serving Totals	371	8	47	16

STEAMED NEW POTATOES

Preparation time: 35 minutes

2 new potatoes (3½ ounces)   1 tablespoon minced parsley

Steam potatoes for 30 minutes. Sprinkle with parsley.

	CAL	CHO	PR	F&O
Recipe Totals	152	34	4	0
Serving Totals	76	17	2	0

HEARTS OF PALM SALAD

Preparation time: 15 minutes

7 ounces hearts of palm,   ¾ cup sliced mushrooms
  sliced lengthwise   (10 small or 4 large)
½ cup watercress (1 ounce)

DRESSING

2 tablespoons no-oil dressing   ¼ teaspoon salt
½ teaspoon sherry vinegar   ⅛ teaspoon pepper
½ teaspoon Dijon mustard   2 tablespoons chives

In a quiche dish (or something similar) layer hearts of palm, then watercress, and top with mushrooms. Combine all dressing ingredients and pour over salad. Cover with plastic wrap and marinate for 1 hour, or toss and serve immediately.

	CAL	CHO	PR	F&O
Recipe Totals	99	21	8	1
Serving Totals	50	11	4	1

BROILED ORANGE

Preparation time: 10 minutes

1 large seedless orange

Cut orange in half crosswise. Section with a grapefruit knife. Place each half in a crimped foil cup with the cut side exposed. Slide under broiler about 2½ inches from heat for 1 to 2 minutes.

	CAL	CHO	PR	F&O
Recipe Totals	73	18	1	0
Serving Totals	37	9	1	0
Daily Totals	1842	153	148	57
Totals Per Person	921	77	74	29

SHOPPING LIST
DAYS 4, 5, 6

Canadian bacon (4 oz.)
lox or smoked salmon (3½ oz.)
Cornish hens (2) (22 oz. each)
lobster tail (14 oz.)
veal chops with bone (2)
   (1 pound)
   (¾-inch thick)
eggs (8)
goat cheese (3 oz.) or feta
   cheese (4 oz.)
plain low-fat yoghurt (1¼ cups)
   (12 oz.)
grapefruit (1)
apple (1) (5½ oz.)
lemon (1)
raspberries (2 baskets) (or
   frozen, unsweetened)
escarole (2 oz.)
watercress (½ oz.)
red potatoes (4) (3½ oz. each)
green beans (11 oz.)
cabbage (7 oz.)
cucumber (½)
fennel (10 oz.)
Belgian endive (7 oz.)
spinach (2 bunches)
tomato (1 medium)
chives (1 bunch)
red pepper (1)

green pepper (1)
parsley (1 large bunch)
mushrooms (10 small or 4 large)
wheat Lahvosh (1 box)
baguette (2 oz.)
enoki mushrooms (1 pkg.)
   (2 oz.)
Angostura Bitters (optional)
white wine (9 oz.)
Dijon mustard
olive oil (smallest quantity
   available)
diet ginger ale (1 can) or
   champagne (1 split) (13 oz.)
tomato juice (1 can) (12 oz.)
beef bouillon (1 can, full-
   strength) (10½ oz.)
   (or homemade)
chicken stock—Swanson's
   (2 cans) (14½ oz. each)
   (or homemade)
hearts of palm (1 can) (15 oz.)
cream of tartar
salt
pepper
caraway seeds or poppy seeds
paprika
garlic clove (1)

DAY 7—SUNDAY

Brunch

Wheat Lahvosh with Caviar

Caviar Omelette

Dinner

Turkey Scallopini with Cannellini Beans

Steamed Broccoli

Teahouse Salad

Broiled Pink Grapefruit

Brunch

2 wheat Lahvosh (5-inch diameter) with 1 ounce caviar

	CAL	CHO	PR	F&O
Recipe Totals	192	20	13	6
Serving Totals	96	10	7	3

CAVIAR OMELETTE

Preparation time: 20 minutes

2 whole eggs
1½ tablespoons minced chives
2 egg whites
Pinch of cream of tartar
⅛ teaspoon salt

Pinch of pepper
¼ cup ricotta cheese
(2 ounces)
1 ounce caviar

Put the two whole eggs in a mixing bowl and beat with a whisk. Add chives. In a separate bowl, using a clean whisk, beat the egg whites with the cream of tartar until they stand in soft peaks. Fold the beaten whites into the whole eggs.

Meanwhile, heat a nonstick skillet for 2 minutes over medium heat. Pour in the egg mixture and turn heat down as low as possible. Cover and let rest 3 minutes or until eggs are set. Uncover, and with a spatula, loosen omelette from sides and bottom of skillet. Season with salt and pepper.

Break ricotta cheese into small chunks and sprinkle over half of the omelette. Fold the other half of the omelette over the cheese. Cover for 1 minute to warm the cheese. Divide omelette in half, place on plates, and top each half with ½ ounce caviar.

Note: If you are in a hurry, the whole eggs and egg whites can be beaten together, but this will produce an omelette that is not as fluffy and large.

	CAL	CHO	PR	F&O
Recipe Totals	409	5	39	26
Serving Totals	205	3	20	13

Dinner

TURKEY SCALLOPINI WITH CANNELLINI BEANS
Preparation time: 25 minutes

Rich's white-meat turkey scallops are available nationwide. To make an easy and delicious sauce, Hunt's Special Tomato Sauce and Progresso Cannellini Beans are perfect. If these are not available, you may substitute with other brands, of course.

Purchase 21 ounces of raw turkey scallops or 21 ounces raw white meat turkey cut in ¼-inch slices. Use 14 ounces for this recipe. Place the remaining turkey, single-layered, in sealed foil and bake at 350° for 15 minutes. Cool, then refrigerate for lunch on Day 9.

14 ounces turkey scallops
¼ teaspoon salt
½ teaspoon olive oil
1 teaspoon minced garlic
1 cup Hunt's Special Tomato Sauce

1 cup cannellini beans, rinsed and drained
4 tablespoons dry red wine
½ teaspoon oregano
Freshly ground pepper to taste

Sprinkle turkey with salt. Heat skillet over medium heat for 2 minutes. Add olive oil. Sauté turkey scallops 1 minute on each side. Remove scallops. Add garlic to skillet and sauté 30 seconds. Return scallops to skillet with tomato sauce, cannellini beans, wine, and oregano. Simmer covered 10 minutes. Transfer turkey to heated plates and reduce the sauce. Serve turkey covered with sauce and beans. Add freshly ground pepper to taste.

	CAL	CHO	PR	F&O
Recipe Totals	850	39	122	19
Serving Totals	425	20	61	10

STEAMED BROCCOLI

Preparation time: 20 minutes

3 cups steamed broccoli
    flowerets (frozen or fresh)

Reserve 1 cup of broccoli for lunch tomorrow.

	CAL	CHO	PR	F&O
Recipe Totals	78	14	9	0
Serving Totals	39	7	5	0

TEAHOUSE SALAD

Preparation time: 10 minutes

  8 water chestnuts, sliced
1½ cups bean sprouts
  2 tablespoons chopped
    green onions
  2 tablespoons no-oil
    dressing

1 teaspoon sesame oil
  (Chinese variety;
  not cold-pressed)
1 teaspoon soy sauce
1 tablespoon grapefruit juice
  Scant ¼ teaspoon salt
⅛ teaspoon pepper

Combine water chestnuts, sprouts, and green onions in a bowl. Mix remaining ingredients in a small bowl and pour over vegetables. Toss well and serve.

	CAL	CHO	PR	F&O
Recipe Totals	179	23	10	6
Serving Totals	90	12	5	3

BROILED PINK GRAPEFRUIT

Preparation time: 5 minutes

1 pink grapefruit

Cut grapefruit in half and section. Preheat broiler. Put grapefruit in a piece of foil crimped into the shape of a cup. Broil 2½ inches from heat 1½ to 2 minutes.

	CAL	CHO	PR	F&O
Recipe Totals	80	20	0	0
Serving Totals	40	10	0	0
Daily Totals	1788	121	193	57
Totals Per Person	894	61	97	29

DAY 8—MONDAY

Breakfast
Banana Blend

Lunch
Stobo Castle Salad

Wheat Lahvosh

Dinner
Swordfish en Moutarde

Wild Rice

Carrot Toss

Creamy Baked Apple

Breakfast

Same as Day 2

Lunch

WHEAT LAHVOSH

2 5-inch crackers (1 per person)

	CAL	CHO	PR	F&O
Recipe Totals—Lahvosh	117	19	5	2
Serving Totals	59	10	3	1

STOBO CASTLE SALAD

Preparation time: 20 minutes

1 cup cold steamed broccoli
4 lettuce leaves (any type)
7½ ounces cherry tomatoes
1 can white albacore tuna,
   water-packed, drained
   (7 ounces)

2 ounces feta cheese or
   1½ ounces chèvre
1 tablespoon finely minced
   red onion

BROCCOLI DRESSING

1 tablespoon no-oil dressing
½ teaspoon lemon juice

⅛ teaspoon salt
Pinch of pepper

TUNA DRESSING

3 tablespoons plain low-fat
  yoghurt
1 tablespoon chives
1 heaping tablespoon
  watercress

⅛ teaspoon salt
Pinch of pepper

Combine ingredients for broccoli dressing. Toss broccoli with dressing, divide in half, and arrange on two plates on a bed of lettuce.

Arrange equal portions of tomatoes, tuna, and cheese on the plates.

Place ingredients for tuna dressing in blender and process 15 seconds, scraping down the sides of the blender jar. Pour dressing over each serving of tuna.

Sprinkle each salad with red onion.

	CAL	CHO	PR	F&O
Recipe Totals (includes Lahvosh)	624	41	78	16
Serving Totals	312	21	39	8

Dinner

SWORDFISH EN MOUTARDE

Preparation time: 15 minutes

The amount of mustard called for in this recipe may sound like too much, but you'll be surprised how deliciously subtle it is. This produces a succulent and uncommonly tasty fish.

15-ounce swordfish steak,
  ¾ inch thick (divide in half
  after cooking)
½ teaspoon lemon juice
⅛ teaspoon salt

Pinch of pepper
4 teaspoons Dijon mustard
2 teaspoons minced chives
2 lemon wedges

Preheat broiler for 10 minutes. Rub swordfish with lemon juice. Let stand 5 minutes, then pat dry and season with salt and pepper. Rub one side of fish with half the mustard. Place fish, mustard side up, on a rack in a broiling pan. Broil 3 inches from heat for 3 minutes. Turn fish over, pat dry, and rub with remaining mustard. Return to broiler for 3 more minutes. Test for doneness. Transfer to plates, sprinkle with chives, and serve with lemon wedges.

	CAL	CHO	PR	F&O
Recipe Totals	488	1	78	17
Serving Totals	244	1	39	9

WILD RICE

Preparation time: 1 hour 5 minutes

4 dried shiitake mushrooms
1 cup boiling water

⅔ cup wild rice
1 cup chicken stock

Pour boiling water over the mushrooms and let stand 10 minutes. Remove mushrooms. Strain liquid through cheesecloth and reserve. Place rice in a pot with reserved liquid and stock. Cover and bring to a boil. Lower heat to a slow simmer and cook 50 minutes. Remove 1 cup rice and reserve for lunch on Day 9. Add sliced mushrooms to remaining rice. Heat through and serve.

	CAL	CHO	PR	F&O
Recipe Totals (includes tomorrow's rice)	408	85	24	2
Recipe Totals	204	43	12	1
Serving Totals	102	21	6	1

CARROT TOSS

Preparation time: 15 minutes

1½ cups packed grated
    carrots (6 medium)
  2 tablespoons grapefruit
    juice

¼ teaspoon dill

Combine all ingredients, toss well, cover with plastic wrap, and marinate 30 minutes. This salad can be made ahead of time.

	CAL	CHO	PR	F&O
Recipe Totals	90	20	2	0
Serving Totals	45	10	1	0

CREAMY BAKED APPLES

Preparation time: 50 minutes

  2 baking apples
    (5 ounces each)
½ teaspoon lemon juice
½ cup cranberries, coarsely
    chopped
  2 tablespoons ricotta cheese

⅛ teaspoon cinnamon
⅛ teaspoon grated nutmeg
  4 tablespoons water
    Low-calorie sweetener as
    desired

Core apples and peel on top to a 2-inch diameter. Rub inside and top of apples with lemon juice. Combine remaining ingredients and stuff into apples. Put apples into crimped foil cups and place in water on a baking dish. Bake at 375° for 35 minutes. Sprinkle with low-calorie sweetener, and more nutmeg if you wish.

	CAL	CHO	PR	F&O
Recipe Totals	271	49	4	6
Serving Totals	136	25	2	3
Daily Totals	1869	192	185	40
Totals Per Person	935	96	93	20

DAY 9—TUESDAY

Breakfast

Orange Blend

Lunch

Southwest Special Salad

Dinner

Lamb Provençal

Sonora Salad

Strawberries with Mint

Breakfast

ORANGE BLEND

Preparation time: 5 minutes

1 orange (8 ounces before peeling)
½ cup water

½ cup skim-milk powder
4 ice cubes

Peel orange, break into sections, and remove seeds. Put water in blender. Add skim-milk powder and orange. Process 15 seconds. Add ice cubes and process 20 seconds longer.

	CAL	CHO	PR	F&O
Recipe Totals	200	39	12	0
Serving Totals	100	20	6	0

Lunch

SOUTHWEST SPECIAL SALAD

Preparation time: 15 minutes

1 cup unpeeled apple cut in ½-inch dices (5 ounces)
2 tablespoons grapefruit juice
1½ cups cooked turkey cut into julienne strips ¼-inch thick (7 ounces)

1 cup cold cooked wild rice
½ cup seedless grapes cut in half (3½ ounces or 24 grapes)
4 lettuce leaves
Salt and pepper to taste

Toss apple with 1 tablespoon of the grapefruit juice. Combine remaining ingredients except lettuce and mix well. Toss with remaining juice and serve on lettuce leaves. Season to taste.

	CAL	CHO	PR	F&O
Recipe Totals	764	85	78	14
Serving Totals	382	43	39	7

Dinner

LAMB PROVENÇAL

Preparation time: 30 minutes

4 loin lamb chops (3½ ounces each, without fat or bone)
½ teaspoon rosemary, crushed
½ teaspoon minced garlic
½ teaspoon salt
⅛ teaspoon pepper

1 teaspoon olive oil
2 cups small mushrooms cut in half (20)
7½ ounces zucchini cut into ¼-inch slices
½ teaspoon sweet basil
1¾ cups cherry tomatoes (7½ ounces)

Rub lamb chops on both sides with rosemary and garlic. Sprinkle with half the pepper and half the salt. Heat a nonstick skillet 2 minutes over medium heat. Add olive oil and sauté chops 4 minutes. Turn them over and sauté 3 more minutes. Transfer to a warm plate and cover with foil.

Put mushrooms in skillet and sauté 1 minute. Add zucchini, basil, and remaining salt and pepper. Continue to cook 4 more minutes, constantly stirring and tossing. Add cherry tomatoes and cook an additional 2 minutes. Surround lamb chops with vegetables and serve immediately. Lamb is most delicious when served pink.

	CAL	CHO	PR	F&O
Recipe Totals	703	21	87	29
Serving Totals	352	11	44	15

SONORA SALAD

Preparation time: 10 minutes

1⅔ cups cucumber, peeled,
   seeded, and sliced ⅛ inch
   thick

½ cup red onion rings

DRESSING

3 tablespoons no-oil dressing
2 tablespoons parsley
1 tablespoon chives

½ teaspoon minced garlic
¼ teaspoon salt
⅛ teaspoon pepper

Combine cucumber and onion rings in a bowl. Put all dressing ingredients in a blender and process 20 seconds. Pour dressing over salad, toss well, and serve.

	CAL	CHO	PR	F&O
Recipe Totals	66	14	3	0
Serving Totals	33	7	2	0

STRAWBERRIES WITH MINT

1½ cups strawberries, fresh or
   frozen (unsweetened)

Serve in glass dish and garnish with mint.

	CAL	CHO	PR	F&O
Recipe Totals	84	19	0	0
Serving Totals	42	10	0	0
Daily Totals	1817	178	180	43
Totals Per Person	909	89	90	22

SHOPPING LIST
DAYS 7, 8, 9

Rich's White-Meat Turkey
  Scallops (21 oz.)
swordfish (raw) (15 oz.)
lamb chops (4) (3½ oz. each,
  no fat or bone)
eggs (4)
ricotta cheese (2 oz.)
feta cheese (2 oz.) or chèvre
  (1½ oz.)
plain low-fat yoghurt (¾ cup)
  (6 oz.)
grapefruit (2)
lemon (1)
apples (3) (5 oz. each)
cranberries (½ cup) or lunch-
  pack box of raisins
orange (1) (8 oz.)
chives (2 bunches)
broccoli (1 bunch)
bean sprouts (1½ cups)
scallions (1 bunch)
cherry tomatoes (15 oz.)
lettuce (1 head)
red onion (1)
watercress (1 small bunch)

carrots (6 medium)
mushrooms (20 small)
zucchini (8 oz.)
cucumber (1)
parsley (1 bunch)
dried shiitake mushrooms (4)
wild rice (raw) (⅔ cup)
skim-milk powder
red wine (2 oz.)
Oriental sesame oil (smallest
  bottle available)
soy sauce (small bottle)
chicken stock—Swanson's
  (1 can) (14½ oz.) (or equal
  amount of homemade broth)
Progresso cannellini beans
  (1 cup)
Hunt's Special Tomato Sauce
  (1 cup)
water-packed tuna (1 can)
  (7 oz.)
nutmeg
oregano
dill
garlic (1 small head)

DAY 10—WEDNESDAY

Breakfast

Canadian Bacon

Lahvosh

Hot Virgin Bloody Bull

Lunch

Emerald Soup

Artichoke and Potato Fritatta

Dinner

Sole and Scallops in White Wine

Orzo

Steamed Asparagus

Moroccan Finale

Breakfast

CANADIAN BACON

Same as Breakfast, Day 4

LAHVOSH

2 Lahvosh (5-inch crackers)

HOT VIRGIN BLOODY BULL

Same as Breakfast, Day 4

	CAL	CHO	PR	F&O
Recipe Totals—Canadian Bacon	156	1	24	7
Serving Totals	78	1	12	4
Recipe Totals—Lahvosh	117	19	5	2
Serving Totals	59	10	3	1
Recipe Totals—Hot Virgin Bloody Bull	104	16	3	0
Serving Totals	52	8	2	0

Lunch

EMERALD SOUP

Preparation time: 15 minutes

Must be made one day ahead.

1 cup tightly packed cilantro leaves (2½ ounces without stems)
¾ cup scallions, coarsely chopped

1 sprig parsley
29 ounces chicken broth
2 cups plain low-fat yoghurt
¼ teaspoon freshly ground pepper

Place cilantro, scallions, parsley, and half the broth in a blender. Process 30 seconds. Add yoghurt and blend an additional 15 seconds. Pour into a 6-cup container and whisk in remaining broth. Chill overnight. Garnish with cilantro leaves and freshly ground pepper.

Note: This recipe makes 5½ cups. Divide in half. Have 2 servings now, and reserve the other two servings for lunch on Day 12.

	CAL	CHO	PR	F&O
Recipe Totals (includes Day 12 servings)	307	41	20	7
This Meal	154	21	10	4
Serving Totals	77	11	5	2

ARTICHOKE AND POTATO FRITATTA

Preparation time: 20 minutes

2 whole eggs
2 egg whites
  Pinch of cream of tartar
1 tablespoon minced chives
1 teaspoon olive oil
½ cup frozen artichoke hearts, defrosted and sliced thinly (If you use a canned or bottled variety, drain and rinse well before using)

½ teaspoon salt
¼ teaspoon pepper
⅔ cup red potato, shredded
½ teaspoon thyme
1 tablespoon minced parsley
5 cherry tomatoes cut in half

Beat eggs and cream of tartar until foamy. Add chives and beat. Heat nonstick skillet over medium heat for 2 minutes. Add ½ teaspoon of the olive oil to skillet and shake to coat pan. Add artichoke hearts, toss to coat, cover, and cook 3 minutes, stirring once. Season with ⅓ of the salt and pepper. Remove artichoke hearts and set aside.

    Place remaining oil in skillet. Add potatoes and thyme. Toss, cover, and cook 2 minutes. Season with ⅓ of the salt and pepper. Place artichoke hearts on top of the potatoes. Beat the eggs again lightly and pour over the vegetables. Season with remaining salt and pepper. Cover skillet, turn heat to low, and let fritatta rest 5 minutes or until eggs are set. Uncover, put a plate over the skillet, and invert fritatta onto the plate. Sprinkle with parsley. Divide in half, garnish with cherry tomatoes, and serve.

	CAL	CHO	PR	F&O
Recipe Totals	339	28	24	14
Serving Totals	170	14	12	7

Dinner

SOLE AND SCALLOPS IN WHITE WINE

Preparation time: 20 minutes

½ cup dry white wine
  (4 ounces)
2 tablespoons minced
  shallots (1 large)
7 ounces scallops *PLUS* 11
  ounces scallops for Day 11
  salad
7 ounces sole

2 teaspoons lemon juice
¼ teaspoon salt
⅛ teaspoon pepper
⅔ cup carrots, sliced
  paper-thin
1 tablespoon minced chives

In heavy nonstick skillet, combine 3 ounces of the white wine and the shallots and simmer, uncovered, over medium heat until wine is reduced to a thin film on the bottom of the skillet.

Remove shallots and any liquid; reserve.

Place the remaining wine plus tomorrow's scallops in the skillet. Cover and cook over medium heat 3 to 4 minutes. Remove scallops and set aside for Day 11 salad.

Sprinkle lemon juice over fish and season with salt and pepper. Lay carrots on bottom of skillet and cover with shallots. Lay sole on top and place scallops around the edge. Cover and simmer for about 4½ minutes. Test for doneness. Transfer to warm plates. Reduce pan liquid by half, pour over fish, and sprinkle with chives.

Note: Tonight after dinner, you must prepare the Scallop and Orzo Salad for tomorrow. See recipe, Day 11.

	CAL	CHO	PR	F&O
Recipe Totals	379	26	62	1
Serving Totals	190	13	31	1

ORZO

Preparation time: 25 minutes

Orzo is a small oblong pasta that looks like rice. Ronzoni makes the best domestic version, and it's available in most supermarkets. If you can't find it, you may substitute any small pasta, but I think the twists are the most attractive alternative.

¾ cup Ronzoni orzo, or
    other small pasta
14½ ounces chicken broth
½ cup scallions, sliced
    (1½ ounces)

1 clove garlic, stuck with a
    toothpick for easy
    removal

Place all ingredients in a saucepan. Cover and bring to a boil. Lower heat and simmer very gently for 15 minutes. Turn off heat and let orzo rest, covered, for 5 minutes. Remove garlic clove, discard. Reserve 1 cup cooked orzo for the Scallop and Orzo Salad on Day 11. Divide the remaining orzo in half to serve.

	CAL	CHO	PR	F&O
Recipe Totals	358	69	12	2
This Meal	179	35	6	1
Serving Totals	90	18	3	1

STEAMED ASPARAGUS

Preparation time: 10–15 minutes

12 asparagus spears, fresh or frozen (5 ounces)
¾ teaspoon fines herbs

1 lemon slice, ¼ inch thick
Pinch of pepper
Salt and pepper to taste

Snap tough ends off fresh asparagus. Add herbs and lemon slice to 1 inch of water in a steamer pot (water level should not touch the vegetables). Bring water to a boil. Add asparagus to the steamer basket and cover. Steam for 6 minutes or to desired degree of tenderness. Remove asparagus and divide into two portions. Season to taste. (The herbs and lemon in the steaming water will have added flavor, so you probably won't want to use very much salt or pepper.)

	CAL	CHO	PR	F&O
Recipe Totals	52	14	2	0
Serving Totals	26	7	1	0

MOROCCAN FINALE

Preparation time: 25 minutes

This salad/dessert tastes even better with the addition of orange or rose-flower water. In fact, they add sparkle to almost any fresh-fruit dish.

1 cup chopped radishes (½-pound bunch)
2 tablespoons lemon juice
1 packet low-calorie sweetener (1 gram)
1 orange, peeled and sliced ¼ inch thick (¾ pound with skin)

½ teaspoon orange or rose-flower water (optional) (These come bottled, and you can find them in most Middle Eastern markets and gourmet shops.)

Finely dice radishes. If they taste too strong, sprinkle with 1 teaspoon salt and let stand 20 minutes. Rinse well, drain, and pat dry. Place in a bowl and sprinkle with sweetener and lemon juice. Toss to combine flavors. Slice orange, pouring into the bowl of radishes any juices that run from the orange. Divide orange slices between two plates, top with radishes and, if you choose, a sprinkling of orange or rose-flower water. Serve chilled.

MOROCCAN FINALE	CAL	CHO	PR	F&O
Recipe Totals	103	27	3	0
Serving Totals	52	14	2	0
Daily Totals	1583	188	139	28
Totals Per Person	792	94	70	14

DAY 11—THURSDAY

Breakfast

Strawberry Blend

or

Cranberry Blend

Lunch

Scallop and Orzo Salad

Dinner

Chicken and Artichoke Hearts with Mushrooms

Braised Spinach with Nutmeg

Watercress and Endive Salad

Banana Sidney

Breakfast

STRAWBERRY or CRANBERRY BLEND

Preparation time: 5 minutes

1 cup water
½ cup skim-milk powder
1 cup fresh or frozen
   (unsweetened) strawberries
   or fresh or frozen
   (unsweetened) cranberries

1 teaspoon lemon juice
2 packets low-calorie
   sweetener (use 3 packets
   with cranberries)
4 ice cubes

Put first five ingredients in blender in order in which they are listed. Process on *blend* 20 seconds. Add ice cubes and blend an additional 15 seconds. You may add more water and process further if it is too thick for your taste.

	CAL	CHO	PR	F&O
Recipe Totals	163	32	10	0
Serving Totals	82	16	5	0

Lunch

SCALLOP AND ORZO SALAD

Preparation time: 10 minutes

Must be partially prepared one day ahead

11 ounces cold poached scallops (reserved from Day 10 scallops)
1 cup cold cooked orzo (reserved from Day 10 dinner)

⅓ cup fresh green bell pepper, diced
⅓ cup fresh red bell pepper, diced
4 ounces Bibb-lettuce cups

DRESSING

3 tablespoons no-oil dressing
1 tablespoon lemon juice
¾ teaspoon Dijon mustard

½ teaspoon fines herbs
¼ teaspoon salt
⅛ teaspoon pepper

Combine scallops and orzo in a bowl. In a separate bowl, combine dressing ingredients. Pour over scallops and orzo. Toss to coat. Cover and refrigerate overnight.

Before serving, add peppers, toss. Arrange on lettuce cups.

	CAL	CHO	PR	F&O
Recipe Totals	491	62	54	1
Serving Totals	246	31	27	1

Dinner

CHICKEN AND ARTICHOKE HEARTS WITH MUSHROOMS
Preparation time: 55 minutes

2 large dried shiitake mushrooms

½ cup fresh mushrooms, minced (3 ounces)

14 ounces chicken breast, skinned, boned, and cut in half

½ teaspoon salt

1 teaspoon lemon juice

4 teaspoons red onion, minced

½ teaspoon fines herbs

Garnish: ½ cup defrosted artichoke hearts sliced ¾ inch thick (3.5 ounces) (If you use canned or bottled variety, drain and rinse well before using)

½ teaspoon garlic

⅛ teaspoon each fines herbs and pepper

Boil ½ cup water. Add shiitake mushrooms. Turn off heat, cover, and let stand 30 minutes. Remove mushrooms from water. Cut off and discard tough stems. Mince all mushrooms.

Pound chicken breasts between 2 pieces of plastic wrap, using a mallet or the edge of a plate. Breasts should be approximately 4 inches by 6 inches. Sprinkle with half the salt.

Combine mushrooms, lemon juice, remaining salt, red onion, and herbs. Mix well and divide between chicken breasts. Roll up breasts and place seam side down on a piece of foil 18 inches by 12 inches. Surround the rolls with artichoke hearts sprinkled with garlic. Top with red onion, the remaining fine herbs, and pepper. Seal foil, crimping lightly, and bake at 350° for 35 minutes.

Remove chicken rolls from foil. Slice each into five pieces and place cut sides up in a row on a plate. Arrange artichoke hearts on either side and pour juices over chicken.

	CAL	CHO	PR	F&O
Recipe Totals	459	12	87	6
Serving Totals	230	6	44	3

BRAISED SPINACH WITH NUTMEG

Preparation time: 10 minutes

1 bunch fresh spinach,
   washed, dried, and torn
   (7 ounces)
1 teaspoon olive oil

1 tablespoon sherry vinegar
   Ground nutmeg, salt, and
   pepper to taste

Shake oil in a nonstick skillet to coat. Add spinach, drizzle with sherry vinegar. Cover and cook over medium-low heat 5 minutes. Divide into 2 portions and season to taste with nutmeg, salt, and pepper.

Note: Cooking spinach without water intensifies flavor and reduces need for lots of seasoning.

	CAL	CHO	PR	F&O
Recipe Totals	147	19	12	5
Serving Totals	74	10	6	3

WATERCRESS AND ENDIVE SALAD

Preparation time: 10 minutes

2 cups lightly packed
   watercress leaves (5-ounce
   bunch before cleaning and
   trimming)
7 ounces Belgian endive,
   sliced in half lengthwise

½ cup hearts of palm, sliced
2 tablespoons red onion,
   minced
¼ teaspoon freshly ground
   black pepper

DRESSING

2 tablespoons no-oil dressing
1 teaspoon sherry vinegar
½ teaspoon paprika

¼ teaspoon garlic, minced
¼ teaspoon salt

Divide watercress between two plates. Arrange endive in a spoke design on top of watercress and place hearts of palm in the center. Mix dressing and pour over vegetables. Sprinkle with red onion and ground pepper.

	CAL	CHO	PR	F&O
Recipe Totals—Salad with Dressing	96	15	6	0
Serving Totals	48	8	3	0

BANANA SIDNEY

Same as Day 5

	CAL	CHO	PR	F&O
Daily Totals	1524	180	172	12
Totals Per Person	762	90	86	6

DAY 12—FRIDAY

Breakfast

Soft-Boiled Egg

Grapefruit Half

Lunch

Emerald Soup

Snowbird Salad

Dinner

Choucroute

Gingered Cheese Pear

Breakfast

Preparation time: 10 minutes

2 soft-boiled eggs
  (1 per person)

1 grapefruit, cut in half and
  sectioned

	CAL	CHO	PR	F&O
Recipe Totals	236	21	12	11
Serving Totals	118	11	6	6

Lunch

EMERALD SOUP

Same as Day 10 (use reserved from that day)

SNOWBIRD SALAD

Preparation time: 10 minutes

Chicken must be cooked and refrigerated one day ahead.

1½ cups bean sprouts
  (3½ ounces)
7 ounces cooked, shredded
  chicken
¼ cup scallions, chopped
2 tablespoons soy sauce

½ teaspoon fresh ginger
  root, grated
1 teaspoon Oriental sesame
  oil
1 tablespoon rice-wine
  vinegar
1 lettuce leaf (any type)

Combine all ingredients except lettuce. Toss well. Divide and serve
on lettuce leaf.

	CAL	CHO	PR	F&O
Recipe Totals	419	17	58	14
Serving Totals	210	9	29	7

Dinner

CHOUCROUTE

Preparation time: 45–50 minutes

This is a wonderful dish for a dinner party. Simply increase the ingredients proportionately to your guest list (remember, all our recipes are for two).

We happily include pork in our low-calorie diets. New breeding techniques have made it leaner than ever. In fact, pork compares favorably with skinless chicken in both calories and cholesterol.

If you do not eat pork, you may substitute chicken, or refer to the Emergency Food Plan for other substitutions.

12 ounces boneless pork chops, trimmed of all visible fat
1 pound sauerkraut
1¼ cups onion sliced in ¼-inch rings (5½ ounces)
2 carrots cut in two (3½ ounces)
2 red potatoes, unpeeled, whole (5½ ounces)

2 boiling onions, peeled but whole (2 ounces)
2 tablespoons gin or 4 juniper berries
¼ teaspoon caraway seeds
⅛ teaspoon freshly ground pepper
½ cup dry white wine
¼ cup beef broth

Heat a nonstick skillet over medium heat for 2 minutes. Sauté pork chops 2 minutes on each side. Set aside.

Place sauerkraut in a large strainer or colander and rinse 1 minute under cold running water, tossing it with your hands. Squeeze dry.

Put sauerkraut in skillet and top with onion rings. Put pork chops in the center and surround with carrots. Push potatoes and boiling onions down into sauerkraut. Sprinkle with gin or juniper berries, caraway seeds, and pepper. Pour wine and broth over all and simmer, uncovered, 3 minutes to evaporate alcohol. Cover and continue to simmer 30 minutes, adding a little water after 20 minutes if necessary.

	CAL	CHO	PR	F&O
Recipe Totals	845	74	89	21
Serving Totals	423	37	45	11

GINGERED CHEESE PEAR

Preparation time: 25 minutes

1 pear, sliced lengthwise and cored
½ teaspoon lemon juice
1 teaspoon ginger root, finely grated

2 tablespoons ricotta cheese
¼ teaspoon cinnamon

Preheat oven to 350°. Rub pear halves with lemon juice, then ginger, spreading as evenly as possible. Fill core cavity with cheese and sprinkle cinnamon over entire surface of pear. Place each half in its own crimped foil cup and bake at 350° for 20 minutes.

	CAL	CHO	PR	F&O
Recipe Totals	196	32	5	7
Serving Totals	98	16	3	4
Daily Totals	1850	151	166	56
Totals Per Person	925	76	83	28

SHOPPING LIST
DAYS 10, 11, 12

sole (7 oz.)
scallops (18 oz.)
pork chops (2) (12 oz.)
  (raw, no bone, no fat)
chicken breasts (3) (7 oz. each)
  (no bone, no skin, no fat)
eggs (4)
ricotta cheese (8 oz.)
plain low-fat yoghurt (3 cups)
  (24 oz.)
pear (1)
lemon (4)
banana (1) (6 oz.)
orange (1)
ginger root (small piece)
spinach (1 bunch)
asparagus spears (12)
radishes (½-lb. bunch)
scallions (8)
shallots (1 oz.)
carrots (2) (6½ oz.)
chives (1 bunch)
cilantro (2 bunches)
parsley (1 bunch)
red potatoes (4) (3½ oz. each)
onion (1 medium)
boiling onions (2) (small)
red onion (1)
mushrooms (3 oz.)
green pepper (1)

red pepper(1)
lettuce (1 head)
Bibb lettuce (1 head)
bean sprouts (3½ oz.)
watercress (1 bunch) (5 oz.)
Belgian endive (7 oz.)
low-cal sweetener (1 pkg.)
  (1 gram)
artichoke hearts (1 pkg.) (frozen,
  bottled, or canned)
shiitake or dried mushrooms (2)
frozen strawberries (or peaches)
  (1 cup)
olive oil (check supply)
sherry vinegar (check supply)
orzo (¾ cup)
white wine (½ cup)
gin (2 tablespoons) (or juniper
  berries)
no-oil dressing (check supply)
soy sauce (check supply)
rice-wine vinegar
chicken stock—Swanson's
  (3 cans) (14½ oz. each)
sauerkraut (1 can) (1 lb.)
beef bouillon—Campbell's
  (1 can) (or equal amount
  of homemade)
hearts of palm (1 can)
fines herbes

7

The Snowbird Emergency Food Plan

The Snowbird Emergency Food Plan is designed to be used *only* in the event of an "emergency." You may opt for these alternate foods when the menu prescribed on the Snowbird Diet is unavailable, or unsuitable because of an allergy or aversion to a particular food.

Specifically, the Snowbird Emergency Food Plan offers convenient alternatives for the traveler or the person who must dine out while on the 12-Day Diet. It is also available to those who may not be able to eat certain dishes on the Snowbird Diet for medical or religious reasons.

When you are traveling or dining out, here are some tips to keep in mind:

- If you phone in advance, most airlines will prepare a low-calorie meal for you, or ask for a 1,000-calorie diabetic diet. They are very simple and plain.
- When ordering in a restaurant, be specific about preparation. Don't be afraid to say:
  "Dry broil."
  "Do not add anything."
  "Put on the plate only what has been ordered."
  "Please put the dressing on the side."

- Eat only the portion you are allowed. Place the rest in a "doggie bag" *before* you begin your meal.
- Take along your own no-oil salad dressing, mustard, or vinegar—any of the taste treats that enhance your meals.
- Never use the restaurant's salad dressing. Either bring your own or stick with a wedge of lemon or use vinegar sparingly.
- The melon, grapefruit, and fresh fruit cup for dessert can usually be ordered from the appetizer menu. Don't spend time looking at the desserts listed. *Ask* for the fruit specifically.

For more information on dining out and traveling, refer to chapter 11, "Living the Snowbird Lifestyle." You will discover dozens of practical, sensible, slenderizing tips.

You may notice that rice, which is a very important staple in the Snowbird Diet, has been omitted from the Emergency Food Plan. With the exception of Oriental restaurants, rice is usually prepared with all sorts of hidden calories and fat. It has been omitted for this reason.

The Snowbird Emergency Food Plan is not intended to be a 12-Day Diet. It is a list of acceptable substitutions for corresponding meals on the Snowbird Diet. Unlike the Snowbird Diet, where the meals are exciting, varied, and interesting, the Emergency Food Plan (out of necessity) offers foods that are rather bland and ordinary. Therefore, eat from the Emergency Food Plan only when you must. Otherwise, stick to the delightful foods on the Snowbird Diet.

HOW TO USE THE SNOWBIRD EMERGENCY FOOD PLAN

Trade only a like meal for a like meal. If you cannot eat the dinner for Day 7 of the Snowbird Diet, you may substitute it *only* with the dinner for Day 7 of the Emergency Food Plan. **Do not** mix and match days. The Snowbird Diet has been carefully formulated to provide maximum nutrition and energy as well as optimal weight loss. Do not disrupt this program by substituting, say, the lunch for Day 9 for the dinner for Day 10.

You must *always* substitute any given meal on the Snowbird Diet with the corresponding meal on the Emergency Food Plan.

DAY 1—MONDAY

Breakfast

(Same every day of Emergency Food Plan)

½ grapefruit *or* unsweetened melon wedge
1 soft-cooked *or* poached egg
½ English muffin *or* 1 slice whole-grain toast (unbuttered)
   Decaffeinated coffee *or* tea

Lunch

4 ounces cold cooked shrimp on lettuce (no-oil dressing, vinegar,
   or lemon wedge only)

Dinner

   Consommé
4 single crackers
6 ounces broiled chicken (no skin)
   Steamed green vegetable
   Mixed green salad with vinegar or lemon wedge
   Fresh fruit cup (unsweetened)

DAY 2—TUESDAY

Breakfast

(Same every day of Emergency Food Plan)

½ grapefruit *or* unsweetened melon wedge
1 soft-cooked *or* poached egg
½ English muffin *or* 1 slice whole-grain toast (unbuttered)
   Decaffeinated coffee *or* tea

Lunch

4 ounces dry-broiled fish with lemon
½ cup peas *or* green beans
1 sliced tomato on lettuce with vinegar

Dinner

6 ounces fillet of beef
½ baked potato
½ cup steamed mushrooms
   Large green salad with vinegar or lemon wedge
   Melon wedge

DAY 3—WEDNESDAY

Breakfast

(Same every day of Emergency Food Plan)

½ grapefruit *or* unsweetened melon wedge
1 soft-cooked *or* poached egg
½ English muffin *or* 1 slice whole-grain toast (unbuttered)
  Decaffeinated coffee *or* tea

Lunch

3 ounces thinly sliced roast beef on lettuce with mustard or
  horseradish
6 cherry tomatoes

Dinner

  Consommé
6 ounces large cocktail shrimp *or* 6 ounces white meat turkey
3 stalks steamed broccoli
  Small boiled potato
  Hearts of palm salad *or* mixed green salad
½ grapefruit

DAY 4—THURSDAY

Breakfast

(Same every day of Emergency Food Plan)

½ grapefruit *or* unsweetened melon wedge
1 soft-cooked *or* poached egg
½ English muffin *or* 1 slice whole-grain toast (unbuttered)
   Decaffeinated coffee *or* tea

Lunch

4 ounces V-8 Juice *or* tomato juice
2-egg mushroom omelette
2 ounces sliced grilled ham

Dinner

6 ounces broiled chicken (no skin)
   Steamed green vegetable
   Small boiled potato
   Green salad
½ grapefruit

DAY 5—FRIDAY

Breakfast

(Same every day of Emergency Food Plan)

½ grapefruit *or* unsweetened melon wedge
1 soft-cooked *or* poached egg
½ English muffin *or* 1 slice whole-grain toast (unbuttered)
  Decaffeinated coffee *or* tea

Lunch

4 ounces cold sliced chicken or turkey *or* 4 ounces
  water-packed tuna
  Lettuce
  Sliced tomato and celery *or* jicama sticks

Dinner

6 ounces lobster *or* crab
½ ear corn *or* steamed artichoke
  Large spinach salad with vinegar
  Fresh fruit cup (unsweetened)

DAY 6—SATURDAY

Breakfast

(Omit if having brunch)

½ grapefruit *or* unsweetened melon wedge
1 soft-cooked *or* poached egg
½ English muffin *or* 1 slice whole-grain toast (unbuttered)
   Decaffeinated coffee *or* tea

Brunch

(Only if you omitted breakfast)

   Mimosa: 4 ounces champagne with 4 ounces orange juice
2-egg western omelette
1 slice whole-grain toast or ½ bagel

Lunch

(Only if you had breakfast instead of brunch)

4 ounces cooked chopped ground steak
1 teaspoon steak sauce
   Green salad with vinegar or lemon wedge

Dinner

1 grilled veal chop
½ baked potato with low-fat yoghurt and chives
   Steamed green vegetable
   Mixed green salad with lemon wedge or vinegar
   Fresh fruit cup (unsweetened)

DAY 7—SUNDAY

Breakfast

(Omit if having brunch)

½ grapefruit *or* unsweetened melon wedge
1 soft-cooked *or* poached egg
½ English muffin *or* 1 slice whole-grain toast (unbuttered)
   Decaffeinated coffee *or* tea

Brunch

(Only if you omitted breakfast)

   Mimosa: 4 ounces champagne with 4 ounces orange juice
4 ounces fillet of beef
   Poached egg on whole-grain toast

Lunch

(Only if you had breakfast instead of brunch)

4 ounces grilled or cold poached fish with lemon wedge
   Green salad
1 slice whole-grain bread

Dinner

6 ounces broiled chicken (no skin)
   Small boiled potato
   Steamed green vegetable
   Spinach salad with vinegar
   Melon wedge

DAY 8—MONDAY

Breakfast

(Same every day of Emergency Food Plan)

½ grapefruit *or* unsweetened melon wedge
1 soft-cooked *or* poached egg
½ English muffin *or* 1 slice whole-grain toast (unbuttered)
   Decaffeinated coffee *or* tea

Lunch

   Consommé
   Chef's salad including a 4-ounce total of any of these:
   cheese, ham, turkey, or white of hard-boiled egg
4 single crackers

Dinner

6 ounces grilled fish
   Broiled fresh tomato
½ ear corn
   Fresh fruit cup (unsweetened)

DAY 9—TUESDAY

Breakfast

(Same every day of Emergency Food Plan)

½ grapefruit *or* unsweetened melon wedge
1 soft-cooked *or* poached egg
½ English muffin *or* 1 slice whole-grain toast (unbuttered)
  Decaffeinated coffee *or* tea

Lunch

  Open-face sandwich including:
4 ounces chicken *or* turkey breast
  Lettuce
  Tomato slice
1 slice whole-grain bread
  Mustard

Dinner

6-ounce lamb chop
  Steamed green vegetable
  Small boiled potato
  Spinach *or* mixed green salad with vinegar or lemon wedge
  Melon wedge

DAY 10—WEDNESDAY

Breakfast

(Same every day of Emergency Food Plan)

½ grapefruit *or* unsweetened melon wedge
1 soft-cooked *or* poached egg
½ English muffin *or* 1 slice whole-grain toast (unbuttered)
Decaffeinated coffee *or* tea

Lunch

4 ounces V-8 Juice *or* tomato juice
2-egg spinach and mushroom omelette
1 slice whole-grain bread *or* toast

Dinner

Consommé
6 ounces poached scallops *or* grilled white fish
Green vegetable
1 plain dinner roll (preferably whole wheat)
Green salad

DAY 11—THURSDAY

Breakfast

(Same every day of Emergency Food Plan)

½ grapefruit *or* unsweetened melon wedge
1 soft-cooked *or* poached egg
½ English muffin *or* 1 slice whole-grain toast (unbuttered)
   Decaffeinated coffee *or* tea

Lunch

6 ounces cold shrimp with lemon wedge
   Lettuce
   Celery *or* jicama sticks
4 single crackers

Dinner

6 ounces Cornish hen, chicken, *or* turkey
   Green vegetable
   Large green salad with ½ tomato and vinegar dressing
   Fresh fruit cup (unsweetened)

DAY 12—FRIDAY

Breakfast

(Same every day of Emergency Food Plan)

½ grapefruit *or* unsweetened melon wedge
1 soft-cooked *or* poached egg
½ English muffin *or* 1 slice whole-grain toast (unbuttered)
  Decaffeinated coffee *or* tea

Lunch

  Stuffed tomato including:
1 tomato filled with
4 ounces water-packed tuna *or* shrimp
  Lettuce

Dinner

  Consommé
6 ounces grilled fish
  Grilled tomato
½ baked potato with low-fat yoghurt and chives
  Spinach salad with vinegar or lemon wedge
  Fresh fruit cup (unsweetened) *or* melon wedge

SUBSTITUTE EMERGENCY MEAL

If no regular foods are available, it is acceptable to substitute a prepared low-calorie frozen entree, such as Lean Cuisine, for either lunch or dinner. While this is not ideal, no harm will be done to your weight-loss effort as long as the entree selected meets the following specifications:

Calories: Not to exceed 300
Carbohydrates: Not to exceed 20 grams (preferably less)
Protein: Not *less* than 20 grams
Fat: Not to exceed 10 grams (preferably less)

In addition, a salad of raw, vegetables should be added to the meal.

PART III

Essentials for Success

8

Put Some Muscle into Your Diet

*Exercise Is a Powerful Force
in Quick, Permanent Weight Loss*

A patient once said to me, "I often have the urge to exercise."
"Wonderful," I said. "What do you do?"
"I usually sit down until the urge passes."

It's no secret that physical inactivity leads to obesity. But did you know that *not* exercising can actually *prevent* weight loss, even if you watch what you eat?

It's true. Diet without exercise rarely succeeds.

How Physical Inactivity Contributes to Obesity

There is definitely a correlation between the amount of exercise a person gets and his or her body weight.

Ever wonder how an obese person can eat less than someone who's slim and yet gain more weight? We know that high blood insulin might be the culprit. But studies indicate that inactivity also has a lot to do with it.

A trim person is in motion more than one who's overweight. It's easier for him to move. He is more comfortable doing physical activity.

The heavier a person gets, the less he or she moves. This is a vicious cycle because the inactivity continues to add to the weight problem. An obese person is slowed even further with each excess pound.

It's easy to understand why overweight people slow down. For one thing, the act of moving takes greater effort. And since they are out of condition, it becomes increasingly difficult for them to move efficiently or comfortably.

Studies show that during the course of a normal day, slim people are far more active. Simple tasks like shopping, housework, errands—any job that requires movement—become more difficult with every pound you gain.

Inactivity is fattening. The less physical activity that's done, the fewer calories are burned. When calories aren't burned, they become stored fat. When the body slows down, it needs fewer calories. So, very often, even when obese people cut down on calories, they still aren't moving enough to burn off what they take in.

Result?

Steady, frustrating weight gain.

Living the Sedentary Life

Keep in mind that each time you do something automatically—whether it's driving a car or chopping onions in a food processor—you are depriving your body of an opportunity to burn off calories.

Sound silly?

Every little bit of energy you expend will eventually add up.

Part of the reason why so many Americans are overweight is that we live a fat lifestyle. When we could walk, we drive. When we could stand, we sit. When we could climb the stairs, we take the elevator.

We rationalize this sedentary system by thinking we are saving time. Saving time is very, very important to us.

But what are we saving it for?

Certainly not our old age. Because we might not have an old age if we don't get moving.

Ever meet a person who insists he just doesn't have time to exercise? It's a common excuse. Most overweight people use it.

But did you ever notice how those same people always manage to find time for eating lunch? Watching television? Shopping?

Anyone who has time to have lunch or watch television has time to exercise.

Exercise is an integral and valuable part of the Snowbird Diet program. You might say it is essential for success.

If you want to lose weight quickly, you've got to exercise. And while quick weight loss may be your primary motivation now, you'll soon discover that exercise offers countless benefits that will help you keep the weight off for good.

Why Is Exercise So Important for Weight Loss?

Exercise ensures that you will lose weight quickly and permanently.

Diet without exercise is dreadfully slow.

Without exercise, there are long plateaus where no weight is lost at all.

Without exercise, progress is so slow that it is discouraging and frustrating—two primary reasons why diets are abandoned.

When exercise does not accompany a diet, calories are not burned quickly enough for visible, steady, encouraging results.

In the first stages of any diet, if you do not exercise, you risk the loss of your lean muscle tissue.

Exercise must be incorporated in the weight-loss plan from the very beginning to ensure that the body does not cannibalize its own muscle tissue.

The object of the Snowbird Diet is to reduce body fat, increase muscle tissue, and produce a healthier and happier person. Without exercise—steady, aerobic, well planned, personalized, varied activity—this goal will be next to impossible to achieve.

To produce long-lasting results, diet and exercise must go hand in hand. Studies indicate that people who diet and do not exercise have a poor chance of keeping off any of the weight. About 90 percent of dieters who don't exercise fail.

Exercise Increases Your Basal Metabolic Rate

Who ever heard of burning up calories while you lounge in front of the TV?

As fantastic as it may sound, you can actually burn calories when you are at rest!

No, it's not some magic over-the-counter potion.

It's one of the wonders of exercise.

When you exercise at the proper intensity for the right amount of time, your basal metabolic rate will be boosted. This means that the rate at which you burn calories *when you are at rest* remains higher than normal even hours after you've stopped exercising. The results are fabulous freebies!

The calories you burn during your workout can be *doubled* while you are resting. The exercise heightens your resting metabolic rate and you continue to burn *additional* calories over the next twenty-four to forty-eight hours.

In other words, if you burn off 300 calories during your workout, and if that workout is done at the right intensity and for the proper length of time, over the next twenty-four to forty-eight hours you will continue to burn off as much as another 300 extra calories. (Increased cardiovascular fitness can also produce a surprisingly more active sex life.)

You cannot afford *not* to exercise.

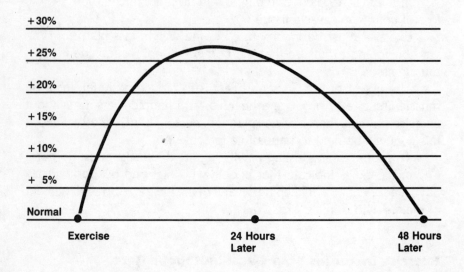

This illustration shows how the metabolic rate rises with exercises. Notice that after forty-eight hours there is still some elevation. This is why exercise can be done every other day and continue to have the desired aerobic effect.

Exercise Reduces Appetite

You've heard people say, "I worked out just long enough to build up an appetite."

That's utter nonsense.

Regular, vigorous exercise does not increase appetite. It *diminishes* appetite.

Once a good exercise program is started, patients notice that their hunger subsides almost immediately. Their natural hunger signals become synchronized with their exercise level, and runaway appetite is kept in check.

This natural phenomenon is a real boost for dieters because it helps them eat less without feeling hungry. Temptation is minimized healthfully without the aid of pills or stimulants.

The longer the exercise program is continued, the better this natural hunger mechanism works.

On the Snowbird Diet, you will be eating smaller portions of highly nourishing food. In terms of bulk, you will be consuming much less than you are used to. Yet, because of your exercise program, you will not feel hungry.

The effects of this diet combined with exercise of the proper duration and intensity will result in the maximum possible *fat loss*, comfortably.

And that's the goal of the Snowbird Diet.

Exercise Can Help Control Binge Eating

We know that exercise reduces appetite. Helping to stop the compulsion to binge is another of its amazing properties.

A person who exercises regularly has less tension, lower levels of anxiety, and fewer bouts with low-level depression, all of which can trigger binging.

Exercise is a way to channel negative feelings into positive action.

When you exercise to fend off impulsive eating, you reap several rewards. Because you are doing something positive, your self-esteem will rise. You will feel more in tune with yourself. You will experience a sense of internal calmness and pride. All these changes in attitude will lead you step by step toward total wellness and fitness and away from binging and depression.

To reap the benefits of exercise, you must do it regularly. Stick to a schedule. Sporadic bursts of frantic, overzealous exercise may do more harm than good.

Consistency is a must.

Exercise Is a Great Way to Cope with Stress

Stress is nothing more than daily frustrations, anger, anxieties, fears, and tensions that have not been expelled. Like steam in a pressure cooker, they build up if not vented in some positive way.

If you do nothing about these feelings—if you internalize them without taking action to vent them—they can be as dangerous to your health as is obesity.

One of the best-known ways to rid your body of these accumulated pressures is to exercise.

Regular workouts are extremely effective at easing the pressure and anxiety brought on by stress.

If you exercise regularly, stress has little chance to build up.

Thus, with exercise you can avoid the health risks associated with stress—stroke, heart disease, high blood pressure, and cancer, to name a few.

Exercise as Part of the Snowbird Diet Can Reduce or Eliminate Major Health Risks

The regular exercise program recommended as part of the Snowbird Diet can reduce or eliminate the major causes of sudden death that strike people in their "prime" years—between the ages of 30 and 60.

Specifically, the number-one cause of death in men in this age group is heart attack. In women, heart attack is the second leading cause of sudden death. (The first cause of death in women is breast and lung cancer.)

Exercise, properly done, increases circulation to the heart. This means that even if some of the arteries are blocked, the blood has more alternate routes it can use to detour the trouble spots.

What this boils down to is that even if you do have a heart attack, this increased blood supply greatly increases your chances of surviving.

Regular exercise appears to increase the level of HDL (good cholesterol) in the blood, which is additional insurance against obstructive heart disease.

Of the eleven major coronary risk factors listed by the American Heart Association, all but one may be either reduced or eliminated with the Snowbird Diet program:

1. *Smoking*
With proper nutrition, stress management, and especially exercise, the task of quitting often becomes easier.

2. *Obesity*
The Snowbird Diet reduces the percentage of body fat and builds lean muscle tissue.

3. *Hypertension or high blood pressure* (over 140/90)
Diet, exercise, and proper stress management are effective for reducing high blood pressure *without* drugs.

4. *Stress*
The Snowbird Diet combines good nutrition, stress management, and regular exercise with effective lifestyle modifications to greatly reduce stress.

5. *High LDL (bad cholesterol) and high triglycerides**
The combination of proper diet and regular exercise reduces bad cholesterol and triglycerides, while increasing levels of HDL (good cholesterol).

6. *Abnormally high blood sugar*
The Snowbird Diet is carefully formulated to reduce blood-sugar levels (by reducing blood insulin).

7. *Oral contraceptives in inactive females, especially those who are over 30 and smoke*

---

*Triglycerides are fats that come from carbohydrates. They are the form in which fat is stored in the body.

The combination of age, inactivity, oral contraceptives, and smoking drastically reduces HDL (good cholesterol). The Snowbird Diet raises HDL and, in addition, helps make it easier to quit smoking by changing an inactive woman into an active, more energetic one.

8. *Diet high in animal fats and cholesterol*
The Snowbird Diet reduces animal fats and cholesterol.

9. *Sedentary lifestyle and inactivity*
A regular exercise program and lifestyle adjustments effectively obliterate this health risk.

10. *Abnormal electrocardiogram or stress test*
This can be greatly improved with the Snowbird Diet's formula for permanent weight loss.

11. *Genetic background*
Alas, this book can do nothing to change your genetic background. But changing ten risk factors of eleven isn't bad.

What Other Health Risks Are Reduced by Exercise?

Hardening of the arteries is caused by plaque buildup in the arteries. Exercise seems to retard the development of such plaque, which in turn reduces the risk of stroke.
Exercise also increases intestinal mobility.
When food moves through the intestines at a slow pace, it risks becoming toxic. When this happens, it often leads to an increased risk of chronic constipation and even cancer.
Exercise increases the speed at which food moves through the system, effectively reducing the risks of toxic intestinal matter.

Exercise Is a Key to Longer Life

Exercise can be a major force in living longer because it can reduce or eliminate most of the major risks of premature sudden death.
The human body responds so beautifully to aerobic activity that

even those who have abused their bodies for years can often reha-
bilitate their health and even *reverse* the degenerative effects of aging.

Unlike a machine that wears down gradually with use, the body
can improve. In fact, the more you use it, the better it gets.

Exercise Can Slow the Aging Process

Along with diet and behavior modification, exercise can be a roadblock
to the process of aging.

Premature aging is, in large part, due to poor living habits
(overeating, inactivity, excessive smoking, et cetera). With the Snowbird Diet, these habits can be altered, and in some cases premature
aging can be reversed.

While chronological age does influence our body's physiological
age, we have found that patients at the Southwest Bariatric Nutrition
Center have actually been able to reverse the effects of unhealthful
living with the proper diet and vigorous exercise. Many become physiologically younger than their years.

Exercise, it turns out, can be a panacea for the ills of contemporary
life.

No matter what your age, it's never too late to make a healthy
comeback. People in their fifties, sixties, and seventies have been very
successful at warding off the devastating effects of chronic degenerative
disease once they began to practice the principles of the Snowbird
Diet.

Exercise Improves the Quality of Life

It might be argued that long life is meaningless if life is not enjoyable.

Exercise is a key factor in making life not only longer but richer
and fuller.

Over time, the cumulative effects of good living habits promote
a sense of well-being and peace of mind. Many experience what can
only be called a healthy high.

Coordination is better. Mobility and flexibility are improved. Circulation is more robust. Energy is heightened. Anxiety, anger, and
depression are reduced. Strength and endurance are elevated. Muscles
are toned and firm. In short, the body and mind are performing at
their peak.

This state of health spills over into other areas of life. Outlook is more positive. Self-esteem is high. There is confidence, calmness, and love of life and increased sexuality that can come only when life is lived at its fullest.

That's what happens when the body is fit and well cared for.

The better care you take of yourself today, the better (and happier) you will feel in the future.

Your life's quality can improve almost immediately with the Snowbird Diet. Do it now. As someone said, "Life is not a dress rehearsal."

Develop a Positive Attitude

One reason why many people can't stick with a good fitness program is that they have a poor attitude.

If you are always looking for an excuse not to exercise, you'll surely find one. But this kind of attitude leads to obesity—not to fitness. It's time to shed fat thinking and get on to a slender life.

So many people have the mistaken notion that exercise is painful or difficult. But it isn't *if* you do it right.

The Snowbird Diet shows you how to improve your physical condition little by little through diet, exercise, and a more positive outlook. You'll soon discover how exercise can be one of the most invigorating, rewarding experiences of your life. It's entirely possible that you will actually look forward to exercise, rather than dread it.

Many people have been put off by exercise because they have tried to do too much too soon. They think their bodies can be shaped up in a matter of days.

What happens when you totally ignore your body's level of fitness?

You push far beyond your current physical limit and usually end up with a serious injury.

And if an injury doesn't sideline you, the frantic pace probably will. Don't start out at a strenuous pace. Start out slowly and build up your endurance gradually. It's healthier and much more rewarding in the long run.

In his book *California Diet and Exercise Program*, Dr. Peter Wood discusses an interesting approach to changing your attitude toward exercise.

Instead of calling it "exercise," which so many people associate with pain and hard work, Dr. Wood refers to exercise as "play."

It makes wonderful sense!

Webster's Dictionary defines *play* this way: "to employ oneself in a diversion, amusement, recreation, or sport."

Adopting this attitude about exercise—thinking of it as play—makes it seem almost like an irresistible adventure. Adventures are chances to try new things, meet new people, set new goals, and make discoveries.

Think what the word *play* meant to you as a child.

You were eager to go out to *play*.

It was something you did regularly, because it was fun.

You invented new ways to play each day. That made playtime more fun and kept you interested.

Actually, playtime included long hours of vigorous exercise—but you didn't think about it then because you were having too much fun.

When you begin to think about exercise in terms of *play*, every encounter with exercise will be fun—a new adventure.

It is surprising how just this little change in terminology can be the turning point in how you view exercise.

Exercise, or "play," will become a daily part of your life. You will look forward to it. You will learn to love it. It will feel good. It will be fun and rewarding.

BABY STEPS TO FITNESS

You've decided to play for fitness. But where do you start?

First you must build a foundation. The lean machine you want to build needs a sturdy, flexible base.

STEP 1: See Your Physician

Before beginning any exercise program, it's wise to have a complete physical examination. This evaluation should include an exercise stress test. The stress test may detect heart problems before symptoms occur.

Based on the results of your complete physical evaluation, your physician may have some guidelines for you to follow in order to exercise at your best.

STEP 2: Set Goals

By giving yourself something to work toward, you can increase your chances for success.

You need to set both short-term goals and long-term goals.

Short-term goals will eventually lead to long-term goals. They should be almost the same as long-term goals, but they should be achievable within a shorter period of time. Include the date you want to reach the goals.

Good short-term goals might be as follows:

1. To walk around the block (by the end of the week)
2. To walk more while in the house (by next week)
3. To take the stairs at work instead of the elevator (in two weeks)
4. To walk one mile (in one month)

Long-term goals should be realistic, difficult, but attainable. Allow a *reasonable* length of time to achieve them, and state your long-term goals in a positive way.

For instance, if you do little or no exercise at the moment, an unreasonable long-term goal would be to run a marathon within three months. That's a sure way to fail. Making goals unrealistic and too difficult will lead only to frustration and disappointment.

On the other hand, a brisk three-mile walk *every day* (in four months) would be a reasonably difficult long-term goal that you could accomplish.

The following chart gives you an idea of how to set up a goal chart for yourself in your Snowbird Workbook.

Be positive about your goals without making them unrealistic. That way you can visualize the way you will look and the way you will feel once you have met your goal. On the other hand, if you state your goal in negative terms, "I will not be lazy and not exercise for two months," it is impossible to visualize yourself other than as lazy and sedentary.

Write them down on your chart.

You need to know where you're going.

And you'll be encouraged when you look back on where you've been.

Making a goal chart will track your physical improvement and your progress. This is an enormously encouraging assignment.

STEP 3: Get Help If You Need It

Let's say you have set your short-term and long-term goals but are not sure what to do next.

My advice is to seek help from a trained, knowledgeable fitness expert. Don't rely on unqualified friends or uneducated, so-called fitness experts to develop your program.

To find a qualified expert, an exercise consultant, or an exercise leader, check with your local hospital to see if it has a health-promotion department. If it does, there will probably be a trained exercise physiologist on staff.

Another resource for fitness guidance is your local college or university. Physical-education departments often have exercise specialists who do private consultations.

Or you might locate an exercise physiologist in the phone book, listed under "Fitness."

While health clubs and exercise studios may be helpful, it's wise to make sure their fitness personnel are properly trained.

For instance, ask if the "expert" has a degree in physical education or exercise physiology. Check to see whether he or she completed a certification program, and ask what type of program it was. If it was only a weekend workshop, the "expert" is not necessarily certified.

Currently there are no national guidelines for certification, and many training programs may claim to be certifiable when in fact they are not.

You Must Play at the Proper Intensity

To get the most out of your exercise, you must play vigorously.

To determine just how vigorously you should play, you must find your *target heart-rate zone*.

This target heart-rate zone can be calculated in two ways:

It can be calculated from the results of your exercise stress test. Your physician or exercise physiologist performing the test can give you these results.

EXAMPLE:

Goal: To increase caloric expenditure and lose 20 pounds by June 15.

Behavior: To exercise every day

Current Level of Functioning: Currently do no exercise (or minimal).

Ideal Level of Functioning: 1 hour per day of walking plus more activity.

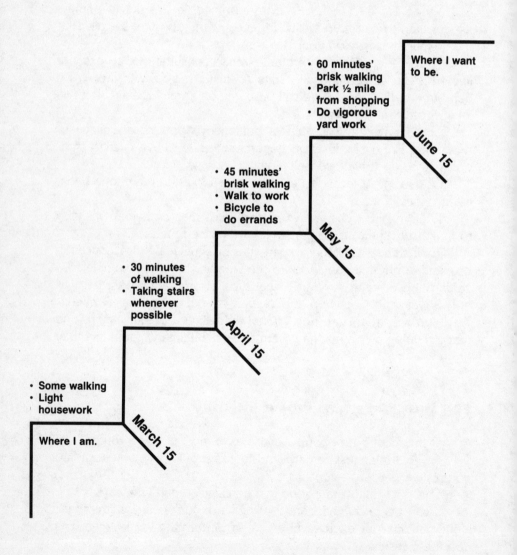

- 60 minutes' brisk walking
- Park ½ mile from shopping
- Do vigorous yard work

Where I want to be.

June 15

- 45 minutes' brisk walking
- Walk to work
- Bicycle to do errands

May 15

- 30 minutes of walking
- Taking stairs whenever possible

April 15

- Some walking
- Light housework

Where I am.

March 15

Develop your program below:

Goal: _____

Behavior: _____

Current Level of Functioning: _____

Ideal Level of Functioning: _____

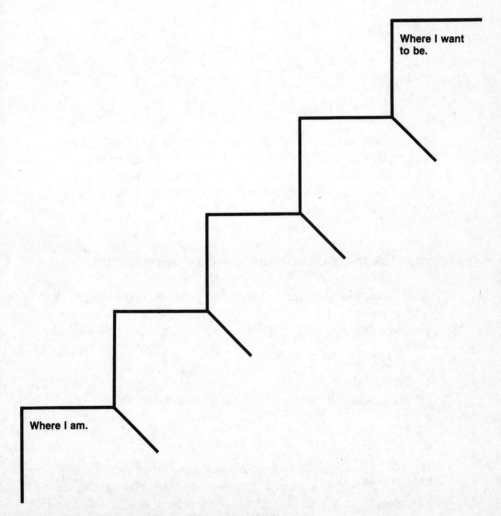

Where I want to be.

Where I am.

Use this chart, or transfer it to your Snowbird Workbook.

Or, it can be calculated based on your age.

The proper intensity for exercise is somewhere between 60 percent and 85 percent of your maximum heart rate.

Here's how to calculate your target heart-rate zone:

1. Subtract your age from 220 (this is a predicted maximum heart rate).
2. Multiply this number by 60 percent, then by 75 percent, then by 85 percent.

Example: age 45

220	175	175	175
−45	× .60%	× .75%	× .85%
175	105	131	149

A beginner should stay in the 60 percent to 75 percent range. Once you are in good condition, you can build up to 85 percent. Averaging 75 percent maximum heart rate is advisable.

However, remember that more discomfort and injuries occur at higher intensities.

How to Put the Target Heart-Rate Zone to Work

Now that you know your target heart-rate zone, you need to practice taking your pulse.

Here are the two most commonly used methods of determining your pulse:

1. *Radial Pulse*
Located near the base of your hand on the thumb side of your wrist.

2. *Carotid Pulse*
Located on either side of your neck near your Adam's apple. *Note:* Don't press hard in this area or on both sides at the same time. Your pulse may respond to the pressure by slowing down.

Count the number of beats you feel during a 10-second period.
Multiply this number by 6.
Another method is to take your pulse for 6 seconds and multiply
by 10, or simply add a 0.

Tips:

1. Memorize the 10-second target-rate-zone values so you
   don't have to multiply by 6 each time.
   For example:

Zone	1-Minute Values	10-Second Values
60%	105 beats	18 beats
85%	131 beats	22 beats

2. Locate your pulse quickly and count within 15 seconds
   after stopping the activity.

3. Exercise at least 3 to 5 minutes before stopping to check
   your pulse.

4. Never use your thumb to feel someone else's pulse—your
   thumb has a pulse of its own.

5. If you are exercising at your predicted target heart-rate zone
   and you feel it is too easy or too hard, **don't ignore how
   you feel.** Adjust your pace accordingly.

6. Certain medications will affect your heart rate. If you are
   taking medications, check with your physician to see if they
   might alter your heart rate.

Explore All the Components of Play

A fitness program is not just stretching, doing 10 minutes of situps or
pushups, and perhaps lifting some weights.

A fitness program is a combination of many components, all of
which affect our bodies differently.

Here are four basic components of exercise for total fitness:

1. *Muscular Endurance*
This is the ability to keep contracting a muscle, or a muscle group, repeatedly, or to contract it over a long period of time. Examples of play that increase muscular endurance are *toning exercises* such as curl-ups, side leg raises, or going through the exercises on a Par-Course in a park.

2. *Muscular Strength*
Muscular strength is defined as the maximum amount of force a muscle or muscle group can exert. Resistive weight training is a basic method to develop muscular strength.

3. *Flexibility*
Flexibility refers to the range of joint motion. It is determined by the ability of the muscles, ligaments, and tendons to move easily without pain through a complete range of movement. Flexibility can be developed by stretching the muscles before, during, and after vigorous exercise.

4. *Cardiorespiratory or Aerobic Exercise*
This is for the efficient functioning of the heart and lungs. It is considered the most important component in a fitness program and is the one that speeds up weight loss. The most delightful activities fall into this category: running, bicycling, swimming, aerobic dancing, brisk walking, and some racquet sports. These types of play use large muscle groups and are continuous and rhythmic.

Find Aerobic Activities That Are Right for You

The following list offers some pros and cons of the most popular aerobic exercises. Perhaps you have health considerations that will eliminate some and endorse others. Try to develop a repertoire of activities that will keep your program fresh, interesting, motivating, and *fun*.

Swimming

Pros

- Involves all major muscle groups
- Offers more total conditioning than do many other activities
- Results in fewer injuries; buoyancy of water reduces excess strain on joints and bones
- Good activity in hot weather

Cons

- Requires efficiency at swim strokes to maintain activity long enough to be beneficial
- Requires access to pool year-round
- Can be a source of ear and eye infections

Tips

- If you do not swim efficiently, you can do dance movements, flutter kick, walk, or jog in the pool to elevate heart rate
- If you have any lower extremity problems or injuries, place a waterski belt around your waist and do continuous leg movement activities in the deep end of your pool

Jogging or Running

Pros

- A convenient activity
- Good benefits in a short period of time
- Level of skill required is low

Cons

- Too much too soon can result in injury
- Negative effect on flexibility
- Activity too intense for beginners

Tips

- Alternately walk and jog until endurance is built up

Aerobic Dancing

Pros

- Adds fun and variety to fitness program
- Can be done with a group, in a class, or at home with a tape
- Uses most major muscle groups

Cons

- If done too strenuously, can lead to injury
- Leaders often push participants too hard
- Some celebrity tapes are relentless and grueling and may result in serious injury

Tips

- Leave out hopping motions to avoid injury
- One foot should always be on the ground
- Build up slowly

Bicycling

Pros

- Enjoyable if you get out and explore
- Not much stress on joints and muscles
- Indoor stationary cycling can be done conveniently at home
- Recommended for both low and high fitness levels

Cons

- Cost of bicycle makes it more expensive than some other aerobic activities
- Indoor cycling takes more effort to get the same result as outdoor cycling. *Note:* Some new models of stationary bicycles include arm-pumping action, which offers better aerobic benefits.
- Outdoor cycling can be dangerous on busy roads
- Bad weather makes cycling dangerous and difficult

Tips

- Join a bicycle club to learn enjoyable routes in your area
- Buy a comfortable seat

Walking

Pros
- Can be done by anyone, almost anywhere, and requires no special equipment except good shoes
- No special skills required
- Injury rate is low
- Aerobic fitness level achieved can be high
- Highly recommended for beginners

Cons
- Takes longer to get same aerobic benefits as more vigorous activities
- Once a person becomes fit, it's hard to walk fast enough to elevate heart rate into target zone

Tips
- Once you are too fit to keep your heart rate elevated by walking, add hand weight (up to 3 pounds per hand) and/or waist weight belt

Roller Skating

Pros
- Research shows that roller skating at a speed of 10 mph is equivalent to jogging a 12-minute-mile pace
- Good social activity
- Exhilarating activity

Cons
- Good skating areas are not always easy to find
- Higher incidence of injury than most aerobic activities
- Must make effort to keep moving continuously to keep heart rate elevated

Minitrampoline

Pros

- Good for those who suffer muscular or bone problems
- Convenient to do in a limited space at home

Cons

- Not as efficient as jogging. Running on a minitrampoline for 30 minutes is the equivalent of running a mile in 12 to 13 minutes.
- Reduces the pull of gravity and therefore decreases the workload. Exerciser's legs are boosted up and therefore over- all workload is reduced.

Sports (Including Racquetball, Tennis, Handball, and Basketball)

Pros

- Fun, challenging
- Adds variety to fitness program
- Opportunity to join league, tournaments, et cetera

Cons

- Stop-and-start activities; actual time that heart rate is elevated into the training zone varies with skill level and competition
- Must rely on having partner(s) to play
- More susceptible to injury

Tips

- Engage in sport-type activity once you are in shape; don't use them to get into shape

Aerobics for the Beginner

Because of celebrity aerobics tapes, you might think aerobic exercises are grueling and exhausting—lots of jumping, kicking, twisting, and wrenching.

Those kinds of exercises might be fine for someone who's already reached a high level of fitness, but for the novice they could—and often do—lead to very serious injury. A body that's been inactive for a long time simply isn't prepared for that kind of strenuous exertion.

The most important thing to keep in mind when you begin any fitness program is to build up *slowly*. Don't be a hero and try to do too much too soon. Total fitness *will* come. But at first you must be patient and take it slowly.

Here are four terrific aerobic activities that work well for the beginner:

Walking
Light swimming or water aerobics
Minitrampoline exercises
Bicycling

None of these requires a high level of skill. Of course, you'll need to learn some basics (especially for swimming), but the initial techniques can be mastered quickly.

All of these aerobic activities can be done for long periods of time, which is great for burning calories. Because of this, weight loss will be accelerated.

Finally, all four of these aerobic exercises have very low injury rates. This is especially important to the novice, who is more vulnerable to muscle pulls and strains.

If you have been inactive for a long time, it's wise to start your Snowbird shape-up with a program that is planned around walking, swimming, minitrampoline exercises, or bicycling. And remember to take it easy.

Fitness Takes Time

There are no shortcuts to fitness. You must take it one step at a time. Be satisfied with slow but steady progress, and rest assured that every little bit really does count.

Some workouts will be more encouraging than others. There will be times when you will notice a big improvement, and other times when you will backslide. When you do regress, remember that it's only temporary.

Think of the body as a bow and arrow. You have to pull far back in order to shoot forward. Temporary setbacks are a normal part of becoming fit. They happen to everybody. Anticipate it, accept it, but don't let it stop you.

Fitness takes persistence. You can't achieve it with an on-again-off-again program. You must be consistent.

It's the cumulative effect of *steady* (not necessarily strenuous) exercise that really counts.

What About Exercise Machines?

Gizmos such as pulley belts, rollers, vibrating tables, and gyrating platforms are a waste of time and money.

In order to burn calories, you must exercise large groups of muscles. This requires good, honest effort. No machine can do it for you.

Letting a machine do the work is passive, not active. When you work out on a passive machine, you are fooling yourself. When no effort is expended, no calories are burned. Fat is not metabolized. You won't lose weight.*

If you don't work at it, the fat won't come off. It's as simple as that.

Can You Spot Reduce?

Many people think that by exercising a certain part of the body they can whittle off the fat in that one area.

It's a lot of bunk!

It doesn't work—it never has. Yet, the misconception persists.

Exercising specific body parts will tone up those muscles. But it will not affect the fat on top of the muscles.

For instance, many people think they can get rid of a roll around their middle by doing sit-ups. If they did 500 sit-ups a day, they would have incredibly hard, toned abdominals. But the layers of fat on top of the abdominals would still be there—soft and flabby.

*Machines such as the Nautilus or Universal are good for muscle toning but not for aerobic exercise.

When muscles are exercised, fat is drawn from *all* parts of the body to meet the energy requirement. Subcutaneous fat does not belong to any particular muscle, nor does it disappear when a muscle is exercised.

If this theory were true, it would stand to reason that people who eat a lot (thereby exercising their jaws and facial muscles) would have thin chins and faces. But the body simply doesn't operate that way.

Will Rubberized Sweatsuits Melt Fat?

Not on the human body. Body fat does not melt like butter in the sun.

The only thing that happens when you wear a rubberized sweatsuit is that your body overheats. It cannot dissipate heat buildup efficiently, which can be extremely critical during strenuous exercise.

This is totally counterproductive to weight loss. When the muscles are overheated, they cannot work at their best.

Exercising in a rubberized sweatsuit in a warm environment is very dangerous. In fact, it can even cause death.

When you exercise, wear clothing that allows the air to circulate freely. Perspiration is the body's best cooling system.

Why Weekend Warriors Won't Win

A patient was explaining his exercise regime to me.

"I can't seem to do much during the week," he said, "but on weekends I really kill myself."

He didn't know how dangerously close to the truth his statement was.

Too often people get into the bad habit of thinking they can wipe out a week's worth of unhealthful living (overeating, smoking, drinking, stress, no exercise) by doing herculean physical activity on the weekend.

However, nothing could be further from the truth.

You can't cure five or six days of overindulgence in a weekend. About the only thing you can do is guarantee that at some point you'll suffer muscle tears, strains, sprains, joint stress, major back problems, and yes, possibly even a heart attack.

Is the answer to take an all-or-nothing approach?

Absolutely not. The answer is to shape up one step at a time at regular intervals throughout the week. It's not only much safer, it's much, much easier.

Being a weekend warrior is simply a bad habit supported by faulty thinking. Now that you know it does no good and is quite possibly harmful, you can begin to adjust your thinking. Don't use the excuse that you haven't time during the week. If you can find time to have lunch, you can certainly find time to exercise.

Remember: slow and steady is what brings results.

Say goodbye to your weekend-warrior thinking.

Why "kill" yourself on the weekend when you can get in shape safely and easily the Snowbird way!

Don't Tackle Too Much Too Soon

Enthusiasm is a fine thing. You'll need plenty of it for success both on the Snowbird Diet and in everyday life.

But don't let enthusiasm lead you to impatience when you are developing an exercise program. Impatience leads to excess, and too much exercise too soon often leads to serious injury or burnout.

Your best plan is to develop physical fitness sensibly and deliberately—one tiny step at a time.

Let common sense be your guide—and ignore the impatient voice that tells you that fitness has come overnight.

Don't be fooled into thinking you are capable of great athletic feats in no time at all. It simply isn't true. You can't erase years of inactivity in five, ten, or even twenty workouts.

The human body will adjust magnificently to exercise if it's introduced gradually.

Following are some guidelines for progress that can be adapted for any aerobic activity.

Note: For maximum weight loss, the recommended duration of any workout is 30–40 minutes, 4–5 times a week. Start slowly and work up gradually to 30–40-minute workouts. Maximum aerobic fitness can be maintained with 30 minutes of exercise, 3 times a week at target level.

Listen to Your Body

If you feel you need to rest during workouts, don't ignore the feeling. Simply slow your pace until you feel better. *Never stop completely or sit down to rest during vigorous exercise.*

Instead, slow the activity to a pace that will allow you to catch your breath and recover your energy. Then pick up the pace and continue exercising.

Warm-Ups Are a Must

You must learn how to warm up properly before your aerobic exercise period. It's one of the most important aspects of a well-developed fitness program.

If you skip this part, you may experience muscle tightness or fatigue during aerobics. Worse, you could end up with a painful muscle pull or strain.

The proper warm-up prepares muscles for aerobic exercise and gradually elevates the heart rate to its target zone.

An ideal warm-up period should last from 3 to 10 minutes, depending on how fit you are and/or the way your body is responding on that particular day. As your physical condition improves, you'll need to spend less time warming up.

Warm-up exercises should not be too demanding. The idea is to charge you up for aerobics—not wear you out.

Develop a set routine for your warm-up period so it will be easy to remember what to do each time.

Suggested Warm-Up Exercises

First do general body movements to stimulate circulation. Do 8 to 10 repetitions of each of these:

1. *Knee Lifts*
Alternately lift knees until upper leg is parallel to the floor.

2. *Leg Kicks*
Alternately kick legs out in front.

3. *Hip Circles*
Place hands on hips and circle hips slowly in one direction, then reverse.

4. *Shoulder Twists*
With hands on hips, twist body to left, turning the head. Then twist body to right in the same fashion. Alternate side to side. It's important to twist *very* gently.

5. *Arm Swings*
Swing arms in circles alternately forward and backward.

6. *Arm Lifts*
Bring both arms straight overhead. Push hands up toward ceiling, coming up on toes.

7. *Shoulder Circles*
Circle shoulders forward several times, then reverse.

Next, do some stretches. Stretch until you feel some tightness, but not until you feel pain. Hold each stretch for 10 to 30 seconds.
Relax all other muscles that are not being stretched.
Keep the body in alignment.
Do not bounce during stretching.
Do not arch or hyperextend the back while stretching.

1. *Side Bend*
Bending at waist, stretch trunk to the right, then to the left. Keep hips centered. Don't allow them to jut out on either side.

2. *Flat Back*
With feet shoulder-distance apart, place hands on thighs and lean forward, keeping your back flat, until you feel a stretch in the back of the upper thighs and in the lower back.

3. *Passive Hang*
With feet shoulder-distance apart, bend over from the waist until your hands are near the floor.

Note: You may bend your knees slightly if your muscles feel very tight.

4. *Side Lunges*
Bend the knee of one leg straight over the toe. Foot should be pointed straight ahead. The other leg is extended straight to the side. Keep both feet flat on the floor. Repeat on the other side.

5. *Wall Calf Stretch*
Stand about 1½ feet from the wall. Place palms flat on the wall. Keeping your heels on the ground, lean toward the wall until you feel tightness in the backs of your legs. Hold. This may also be done one leg at a time.

6. *Quadricep Stretch*
Stand next to wall. Place right hand on wall and grab left ankle behind you with left hand. Push ankle against hand to create a *wide angle between* upper and lower leg. (Don't pull lower leg toward buttocks.) Pull leg back. Hold. Repeat on the other side.

The last segment of the warm-up is to start your aerobic activity very slowly. For example, if you are going to walk, start with a slow walk for about 3 to 5 minutes. Then you can pick up the pace until you reach your target heart rate.

A Cool-Down Is Necessary

Cooling down after aerobic activity is just as important as warming up.

It gradually reduces the heart rate, blood pressure, and respiration rate to resting levels.

Cool-down exercises will also help to remove lactic acid and other waste products that build up during exercise.

When you finish the day's workout, your muscles should be completely relaxed.

Cool-down exercises are almost exactly like warm-ups.

First, finish your aerobic activity period by winding down the pace gradually.

Next, do the same general body movements and stretches that you do in the warm-up portion.

Last, take your recovery pulse to see if it is near your normal resting heart rate. It should be 100 or less.

Muscular Strength and Endurance Training

This phase of the Snowbird fitness program will help you build stamina and strength and at the same time avoid serious injury.

To accomplish this you must do either calisthenics or weight-training exercises.

Concentrate on the main muscle groups:

Upper Body
  Neck
  Arms
  Shoulders
  Upper back
  Chest

Lower Body
  Abdominals
  Lower back
  Buttocks
  Thighs (front, back, sides)
  Calves
  Ankles

Devote equal time to each group. Don't focus on just one or two groups. Remember—spot reducing doesn't work.

As you progress, this segment can fit into your cool-down before stretching.

Following are some basic exercises I recommend for muscular strength and endurance:

Abdominals and Back

1. *Abdominal Curl*
Lie on your back with legs together and knees bent. Feet should be flat on the floor. Start with arms straight up in the air. Slowly roll

head and shoulders off the floor until hands touch knees. Slowly roll back to the floor. Do 2 or 3 sets of 10 repetitions.

2. *Pelvic Tilt*
Lie on your back with knees bent, feet flat on the floor, and hands behind head. Tighten abdominals and buttocks, flattening the small of your back against the floor by rolling the hips. Hold about 6 seconds. Relax. Repeat 10 to 20 times.

Shoulders, Chest, Arms

1. *Wall Push-Up*
Stand about 2 feet from wall. Place palms flat against wall at shoulder height. Slowly bend elbows and bring your face close to the wall without letting your heels come off the floor. Keep back straight. Gently push your body away from the wall. Keep a slight bend at the elbows when arms are extended. Repeat 10 to 20 times.

Legs and Ankles

1. *Semi-Squats*
With feet parallel about 6 inches apart, hold on to the back of a chair for support. Bend knees, lowering body down. Keep back straight. Go down only to the level of the chair seat. Come up slowly. Repeat 5 to 10 times.

Making Calisthenics Fun

Sooner or later, any routine gets boring.

Fight the blahs by constantly inventing new ways to play.

Here are some things my patients have done to turn monotony into something invigorating and delightful:

- Learn a set of exercises for each of the muscle groups, then put them to music. Choose records or tapes that are lively and rhythmic—dance music is always fun.

- Join an exercise class that includes toning exercises. Many people find that the camaraderie and instruction of a good class are invaluable. Some patients have even organized "private" workouts. A few of them get together and hire a professional who gives classes at students' homes.
- Buy an exercise tape or album to follow. Make sure it is not too advanced for you. Some of the popular celebrity tapes are too strenuous for beginners.
- Use exercise stations that are set up in many parks—Par Courses are a good example. This is a fine way to get out in the fresh air, exercise, and enjoy the natural setting of a park at the same time.
- Do toning exercises in a swimming pool. Just being in a pool is refreshing—especially in hot weather. And the water offers additional resistance to make your workout even more effective. Working out in a cool pool can really incinerate calories.

Whatever you do, *have fun*. Play. Vary the activities to keep from getting bored.

When It's Too Hot to Trot

If you're used to exercising outdoors, hot summer temperatures can make things difficult.

This does **not** mean you should stop exercising.

Find out how your body reacts to exercise when the weather is hot, and know your limits.

Anytime the temperature is over 90 degrees, the humidity is 40 percent to 50 percent, or the sunlight is direct and intense, proceed only with extreme **caution.**

Exercising outside under any of these conditions can be deadly.

Instead, plan to exercise early in the morning or in the evening after it cools off. Avoid doing any strenuous activity during the heat of the day.

And remember to drink plenty of water. Drink more than normal if you are perspiring a lot.

Another solution for hot-weather fitness is to switch to a type of exercise that can be done indoors.

Walk in a cool shopping mall.

Ride a stationary bicycle.

Go swimming—the perfect summertime exercise. Working out in a pool is a marvelous summer refreshment.

Again I stress, **drink plenty of fluids.** Water is best. Remember that in hot weather you can lose as much as 3 quarts of critical body fluid *per hour.* So, get into the habit of drinking water every 10 or 15 minutes during exercise and plenty before and after the workout.

Remember that a pint of water weighs one pound. Therefore, if you are down 2 pounds after a workout you must replace that lost fluid by drinking 2 pints of water. Don't make the mistake of thinking you've lost 2 pounds of fat. Fat doesn't disappear that quickly. You have lost water, and in summer temperatures your body desperately needs to replace it.

For a refresher course on water, reread chapter 4, "Wondrous Water." Review it as often as necessary until you understand it and it becomes part of your life.

Your body will perform at its best only when it is fully hydrated.

Wear the Right Clothes

Having the right clothing for exercise is important. You must be able to move freely—feel cool, comfortable, and unrestricted.

When the weather is chilly, dress in a few thin layers rather than in one heavy, bulky garment.

Select garments of 100-percent cotton to wear next to your skin. Cotton absorbs perspiration best and lets your skin breathe. Never wear too much clothing or your body will be in danger of overheating.

If you join an aerobics class, it's best not to rush out and buy tights, leotards, and leg warmers at the beginning. They'll probably make you overheat because so much body surface is covered.

Once you are in better physical condition, your body will be more efficient at cooling itself. Then you might be able to wear layered, form-fitting exercise clothes.

In hot weather wear light, loose clothing. Cotton is great because it's cool. Expose as much skin as possible. **Never** wear sweatsuits or slacks when you exercise in hot weather.

How to Choose Shoes

For walking, jogging, and sports, the correct shoes make a big difference.

First, they will ensure comfort. Better, they are designed to reduce injury.

Fine, well-made athletic shoes are expensive. But a better investment is hard to find.

For aerobics, select shoes that have plenty of support and cushioning in the arches and heels.

Go to a store that specializes in athletic shoes. Their salespeople are trained to help you find and fit the right shoes for you.

Because there are so many different types of shoes today, you are bound to find a pair that seems tailor-made for your feet. It's best to try them on with the type of socks you will be wearing for exercise. Move around the store in the shoes for several minutes before you decide to buy.

Having the proper shoes can make or break exercise—especially if you are a tenderfoot.

Every Little Bit Counts

Little by little, every bit of energy you exert will eventually add up to pounds lost. If you have lost all you want, exercise will make maintenance a breeze.

Your goal overall should be to dump your old sedentary lifestyle and become a more active, energetic person.

Regular exercise is one of the best ways to achieve that goal. In addition to structured exercise, there are dozens of ways to burn calories and live a more active daily life.

Following is a list of some painless ways to boost your energy output. I'm sure you'll be able to think of dozens more that apply to your lifestyle.

- Walk to and from work.
- If it's too far to walk, drive part of the way and walk the rest.
- Take stairs every opportunity you get.
- Do your housework and yard work energetically.

- Shun automation—doing things manually burns calories.
- Make it a habit to park at the far end of parking lots.
- Do your errands on foot.
- Take every opportunity to carry, lift, bend, and push.
- Take walking breaks instead of coffee breaks.
- When you travel, see the sights on foot.
- When you are delayed at an airport, take a brisk walk from one end of it to the other.
- When sitting, circle the ankles and point and flex the feet.

Motion Motivation

Many people have trouble sticking with a fitness program. They let it become dull or boring. They do it halfheartedly. They have the wrong attitude. They find excuse after excuse.

But excuses lead to the fat farm.

And that's not where you're going.

You are now on the road to self-esteem, health, fitness, and freedom.

You have discarded excuses in favor of action.

Here are some ways you can reinforce your commitment to an active lifestyle:

- Invest in good exercise clothing and proper shoes. Nothing motivates like dollars spent.
- Chart your progress. Keep records in your Snowbird Workbook of all your improvements, no matter how small.
- Take your measurements so you will know exactly how many inches in all you have lost.
- Think of exercise as **play**.
- Don't exercise so intensely that you are in pain.
- Add variety and excitement to your program. Do exercises that are fun.
- Listen to music or watch television while exercising, or work out with a friend for a change of pace.
- Be consistent. Don't have an on-again-off-again program. It is psychologically defeating and physically dangerous. Work out a steady schedule and stick to it.

- Become immersed in fitness as a way of life. Read books and articles on fitness. Take classes. Subscribe to magazines. Make it a permanent part of your new lifestyle.
- Exercise socially. Perhaps you can organize a group of friends or co-workers who also want to shape up. A group can be motivating and supportive.
- Develop a support system. Make sure at least one positive person knows what you are out to accomplish. Tell them your goals and ask for their support and encouragement.
- Find a new reason each day to be proud of yourself. Write it in your Snowbird Workbook. Refer to your list as often as you like. Develop a positive attitude toward yourself, toward fitness, and toward life.

Fit? Don't Quit!

Hippocrates said it best: "That which is used develops, and that which is not, wastes away."

This is especially true of the human body.

The more you use it, the better it works.

If you live an active life, not only will you maintain your weight loss, but your physical condition will continue to improve.

The road to physical fitness is a road without end. It leads only to another horizon of health and happiness.

It is ongoing.

It is lifelong.

It is sustaining.

It is the only road to travel.

Stress Management

Exercise is an excellent method of reducing stress and depression as well. The physiological and psychological energy it requires, the increased endorphin production, and the sense of "being in charge" it creates when you are in control of your own body movements combine to produce feelings of well-being in most people.

Stress, in itself, isn't always bad for you. Most college students will perform better on an exam when pressure exists. Stress, especially in moderate doses, can be motivating.

Stress in the extreme can be lethal. High blood pressure, heart attacks, migraines, loss of sleep, poor concentration, ulcers, and colitis can often be made worse by high stress factors.

Binge eating or "nervous eating," so often the downfall of the dedicated dieter, can easily become an addictive tranquilizer for the all-too-common strains of contemporary living.

Learning to take "time out" for yourself with relaxation, whether it's practicing meditation, yoga, listening to music, reading, or enjoying hobbies is no longer a "frivolous leftover" in application of this culture's work ethic but a *necessity* for maintaining your physical and mental health.

At the Southwest Bariatric Nutrition Center, we include deep muscle relaxation combined with positive imagery and "self-talk."

Begin by lying on a couch, the floor, or sitting in a comfortable chair. Turn your attention first to your toes and feet imagining them to feel warm, light, and tingly. Progress upwards, concentrating on your legs, stomach, arms, neck, and every facial feature until your whole body feels light and relaxed. Then practice seeing yourself as you want to look, front, back, and sideways, followed by self-affirmations such as "I am improving every day," "I'm taking control, one day at a time," "I don't need to be perfect," or "I like myself." Relaxation in this way also improves your self-image, and makes you more open to positive suggestions.

9

Positively Slender
How to Think and Act Like a Thin Person

Most overweight people are so obsessed with their appearance that they overlook one very important point. Excess weight is not the problem. It is only a symptom.

The real problem is not external. It is internal. Negative thoughts and feelings inside result in overweight outside.

When you go on a crash diet, it's like putting makeup on a dirty face. The problem is only masked temporarily.

But the Snowbird Diet is able to achieve lasting results because it treats weight problems from the inside out. It teaches you how to become thin in your mind.

Changing a lifetime of negative thinking takes more than a quick crash diet.

It requires a thoughtful, conscious effort to expose subconscious behavior. Then you replace the harmful behavior with new, positive actions.

It's very simple.

Negative thoughts produce negative results.

Positive thoughts produce positive results.

From now on, ferret out all the negative, fattening thoughts and actions that contribute to your weight problem. And work to change them, one by one. Like knots in a tangled ball of yarn, some will be easy to unravel, while others will take patience and persistence.

Fat Is Off!

At the Southwest Bariatric Nutrition Center we have developed a thorough, multifaceted approach that helps patients break out of their negative, fat thinking. Little by little, they learn to think positive thoughts and take positive action.

We call this program FAT IS OFF!*

FAT IS OFF! is an acronym that stands for each of the components of the program:

Feelings
Actions
Thoughts
Imagery
Sensations
Others
Fitness
Forever!

Each of these words represents a special and powerful tool to help you become thin from within.

With FAT IS OFF! you will learn how to pinpoint subconscious eating problems and expose the forces behind them.

You will learn how to come to grips with many of the negative thoughts and feelings you have literally been swallowing.

And you will learn how to deal with your eating in ways that will ensure slenderness now and forever.

1. Feelings

One reason why people overeat is that they have learned to deal with their feelings inappropriately. Namely, they eat.

Instead of taking suitable action in response to boredom, anxiety, anger, loneliness, depression, fatigue, or even happiness, they have learned to bury these feelings with food.

Feelings, then, become *paired* with the urge to eat. In other words, a feeling becomes so intertwined with the act of eating that whenever the feeling surfaces, it automatically triggers the desire for food.

*Adapted from A. Lazarus, *Multimodal Behavior Therapy: Basic ID.*

Clearly, eating is an inappropriate response to any feeling except that of true nutritional hunger. But for many overweight people, eating is much more than a way to provide physiological sustenance. It has become a way of coping with all sorts of unrelated feelings.

Here are some examples.

Martha receives a promotion at work. She is very excited and happy. She equates the feeling of happiness with eating. Her feelings of elation are psychologically *paired* with the urge to eat. Instead of celebrating her promotion in a more fitting way, Martha goes on an eating binge.

Another of Martha's "green lights" is the feeling of anger. When she has a fight with her mother, instead of expressing her anger appropriately, she turns to food. The food buries the anger temporarily, but the eating binge is soon followed by feelings of guilt, depression, and more anger. Martha is compelled to eat more and more.

Like most people, Martha probably has no idea what triggers her uncontrollable desires for food. She probably thinks she has some hopeless character flaw. She may feel depressed because she is "weak-willed" or out of control.

When feelings are paired with a desire to eat, spontaneous binging often occurs. Following a binge there is often deep depression, remorse, and a sense of hopelessness. These negative feelings trigger another binge. And the cycle is perpetuated.

This vicious emotional eating cycle looks like this:

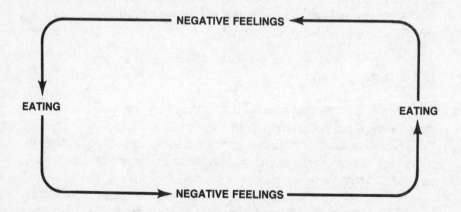

To break this fattening cycle, you must first discover which of your feelings, if any, are paired with eating.

Monitoring Your Urges for Splurges

How can you discover what your own eating "green lights" are? Follow this procedure:

The next time you want to eat, take a moment to decode your true feelings. Write the answers to the following questions in your Snowbird Workbook:

1. When did I last eat?
2. What food do I want?
3. Is this hunger or appetite?
4. When I first felt like eating:
    a. Where was I?
    b. What was I doing?
    c. What was I thinking?
    d. What was I feeling?

Here is how answering these questions can help you get to the root of your desire for food. This example was taken from the workbook of a patient:

1. When did I last eat? *Lunch, two hours ago.*
2. What food do I want? *Doughnuts and coffee.*
3. Is this hunger or appetite? *Appetite.*
4. When I first felt like eating:
    a. Where was I? *In my office.*
    b. What was I doing? *Sitting at my desk.*
    c. What was I thinking? *Daydreaming about a vacation.*
    d. What was I feeling? *Tired.*

By answering these questions, the patient was able to discover the feelings behind his urge to eat.

Since he ate lunch two hours before, he knew the craving for food was not physiological. His body did not require any food.

His desire for junk food confirmed that he was indeed having an appetite attack. Remember, when people are truly hungry, they are more apt to desire good, substantial food, not junk food.

By answering questions 1 and 2, the patient was able to deduct that he was experiencing appetite, **not** hunger.

His answers to question 4 reveal the feelings behind his urge to splurge.

The fact that he was daydreaming might suggest that he was bored or fatigued. He lacked mental concentration.

Finally, he was able to pinpoint the feeling of tiredness.

By continuing to decode his desire for food over the following weeks, he came upon a startling realization. Each afternoon at about the same time, he noticed a pattern of feeling fatigued and mentally fuzzy. He realized that he was experiencing an afternoon slump.

It comes as no surprise that he also had an appetite attack at the same time. When people are fatigued, they are more vulnerable.

His craving for sugar and caffeine was a subconscious way of coping with his feelings. Fatigue and boredom had become paired with his urge to eat.

Because he monitored his cravings, he was able to decode them. Through trial and error, this patient was eventually able to change his fattening behavior.

He began to plan ahead for the afternoon slump. First, he made a list of alternatives to eating. These included taking a walk, making a phone call, reading a magazine, or straightening out a desk drawer. Whenever he had an appetite attack, the list offered immediate ideas on how to cope. This spared him the trying task of dredging up self-control and creativity during the time of day when he was most vulnerable.

To minimize his natural "down time," he started eating lighter lunches. He also began spending half his lunch break walking briskly and breathing deeply.

He planned hourly breaks during the afternoon for stretching and deep breathing.

He kept a supply of harmless snacks on hand (vegetable sticks, low-calorie drinks, sugarless mints).

Ultimately, this patient was able to break out of the destructive eating cycle that had contributed to his weight problem.

Notice: He did not treat the appetite. Recognizing that it was not true hunger, he set about to treat the feelings *behind* the appetite.

In order to change your bad eating habits, you must monitor your feelings and decode your urges for splurges just as this patient did.

Then, take appropriate **action.**

2. Action

Becoming aware of feelings that trigger eating is a step in the right direction. But awareness alone may not be enough to help you make permanent changes.

To make lasting changes in behavior, you must take positive action. For example, if boredom triggers your desire for food, think of ways to eliminate boredom.

Boredom, or any other negative feeling, will not go away by itself. Take action against it.

Start by compiling a list called *Alternative Actions* in your Snowbird Workbook. Include activities you think will help you counteract the feelings behind your eating. List only the things you genuinely enjoy doing. If your list is a bit short, this is a great opportunity to try some new activities. (Some suggested activities are listed later in this chapter.)

Add new alternative actions to your list whenever you can. Try to make them as versatile and exciting as possible. Refer to the list often.

Instead of turning to food, erase the feeling behind it with a rewarding activity. Keep the list with you at all times—you never know when an appetite attack will strike.

The moment you begin to channel your negative feelings into positive action, you will experience a wonderful sense of satisfaction. Realizing that your bad subconscious habits can be broken will be exhilarating and encouraging.

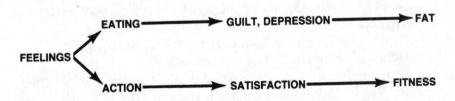

Stop Swallowing Your Feelings

It's important to stop pushing down feelings with food. Swallowing your feelings may seem like the path of least resistance, but in reality it is a destructive, life-threatening behavior.

From now on, find ways to let out your feelings constructively. Following are some positive ways to express feelings:

If you feel tired, get some rest, exercise, or change your pace.

If you feel lonely, phone or visit a friend, make a new friend, or devote some time to helping others.

If you feel depressed, seek professional counseling.

If you feel happy, celebrate with hugs, kisses, conversation, shopping, attending a concert, or having a professional massage.

There must be hundreds of other actions you can add to your list.

Learn to Motivate Yourself

Motivation is one of the most difficult things to instill in another human being. I can't do it for you. No one can. Take the responsibility for motivating yourself.

But what if you just don't feel motivated?

Let me point out that feelings are the *last* to change. If you change your actions first, your feelings will follow suit.

Even if you aren't motivated right now, by taking positive action despite the way you feel, you can develop motivation. Here's an example:

A good way to work yourself out of a depression is to do something constructive. Clean out a closet, organize a file, rake the yard. Do something physical that will give you a sense of accomplishment in a relatively short period of time.

Don't sit around waiting for motivation to strike. Make it happen by taking action.

Remember: Positive action leads to positive results.

Here's another way to take positive action:

Start another list in your Snowbird Workbook. Call it *Why I Want to Lose Weight*. Include all the reasons you can think of for becoming slender and fit.

Keep adding to the list. Read it regularly.

When your goal is clouded by the urge to eat or cheat, read this list to bring it back into focus.

Review *Why I Want to Lose Weight* at night before you go to sleep and in the morning before you start your day. It will do wonders to keep you on the right track.

Your list might include the following reasons:

1. Will look better in clothes
2. Will feel more comfortable
3. Will be more outgoing
4. Will have more energy
5. Will look younger and healthier
6. Will be more attractive

Keep this list handy in your workbook from now on. It is a powerful self-motivating tool.

Learn to Reward Yourself for Good Behavior

Until now, you may have been using food as a kind of reward. Food tastes good. It provides instant gratification. And food can even be used as a tranquilizer.

Your task now is to find new, more exciting ways to reward yourself.

Discover all the things that make you feel good without resorting to food.

For example, when you successfully avoid an eating binge, reward yourself for the positive behavior. Treat yourself to a movie, a new book, a pedicure, or a long, luxurious bubble bath.

In your Snowbird Workbook, start a list called *Rewards for Good Behavior*.

Like the other lists, include only things you really like.

Divide the list into two columns: *Short-Term Rewards* and *Long-Term Rewards*.

Short-term rewards include small pleasures that can be earned with each little victory over eating. A long-stemmed rose for your nighttable is a good example.

Long-term rewards come when more difficult goals are achieved. They should be more elaborate, such as a weekend at a lovely resort or a new outfit after you've lost 10 or more pounds.

Don't Take On Too Much Too Soon

As you become aware of behavior changes you need to make, add them to a list called *Old Habits I Will Change*.

Don't try to change them all at once. Work on them one at a time.

For example, if you have trouble with snacking while watching television, work on changing that habit exclusively. Concentrate on finding alternative actions for that one problem. Focus on the steps you need to take to eliminate old thinking. When that problem is under control and you feel comfortable with having mastered it, then you can tackle another self-defeating behavior.

If you make the mistake of trying to change too much too soon, you'll risk ultimate failure. The mountain is just too big and discouraging.

I can't stress this enough. Don't let impatience lead you to failure. It's taken you a long time to develop your self-defeating habits. Don't expect to erase them overnight.

3. Thoughts

We know it's possible to change negative feelings with positive actions. Now let's explore some ways to change negative feelings with positive *thought*.

The power of positive thinking is a very real precept; it has worked miracles for many, many people. And positive thinking is of particular importance to the dieter.

How does positive thinking change negative feelings?

Remember that feelings are the last to change. Change your thoughts first, and a change in your feelings will eventually follow.

For example, if you say, "I'll never lose weight," that's negative thinking. Tell yourself this negative thought often enough and you'll come to believe it. It will make you feel discouraged and unmotivated.

On the other hand, if you think something positive, such as, "I will lose weight," it will become part of your belief system. If you begin to think positive thoughts, even though you may not believe them now, eventually you *will* believe them. Just as negative thinking produced negative results, positive thoughts will bring positive results.

A positive outlook can indeed change your feelings.

Developing an optimistic outlook will go a long way to ensure the success of your diet. To succeed, you must learn to believe in yourself.

In your Snowbird Workbook, start a list called *Positive Thoughts for the Day.*

Add at least one positive thought each day.

Include positive thoughts you receive from others, such as compliments and words of encouragement (even if you don't believe them).

Read the list often.

Perfectionism Is Poison

One common mistake is equating positive thinking with perfectionism. The fact is, the two are complete opposites.

Perfectionism is destructive.

Perfect behavior and perfect eating are impossible to sustain.

Don't set up unrealistic standards for yourself. It will set you up for failure. Perfectionism fosters negative thinking and negative results: "I might as well eat all the cookies since I already blew it by eating two."

Instead of whipping yourself for being human (and therefore fallible), begin to embrace your mistakes as wonderful opportunities to learn more about yourself. Learning from mistakes is one way to make them work *for* you.

Learn from Your Mistakes

Accept the inevitable. You, like all other human beings, will make mistakes. But mistakes are no longer going to be negative. You are going to learn how to make them rewarding and beneficial.

At the Southwest Bariatric Nutrition Center we have developed a four-step formula to help you. We call the formula the **Hindsight-Foresight** method.

By scrutinizing mistakes in hindsight, we can develop the foresight to avoid similar mistakes in the future.

Here's how it works:

1. When you make a mistake and eat something unplanned, avoid punishing yourself by using positive self-talk. Instead of saying,

"I just blew another day of dieting with that piece of cake," comfort yourself with positive thoughts: "It's okay to make mistakes. Everyone does. I'll learn to do better next time."

2. Monitor and decode your thoughts, actions, and feelings to determine what motivated the mistake. Use your notebook.

3. Decide how a similar mistake can be avoided in the future. Prepare yourself for next time, and learn to act **before** you eat.

4. Let go. Forgive yourself and get on with your diet. A little mistake doesn't have the power to stop you!

Life Is Never Fair

The sooner you embrace this thought, the easier it will be for you to come to terms with life's inequities.

Don't get mired in the quicksand of thoughts such as, "It's not fair. She eats anything she wants and never gains weight." Or, "Why should I be the one to have this problem?"

Life isn't fair to anyone. Everybody has a burden whether it's apparent to you or not.

Many people must live a lifetime with their afflictions, but yours is something that can be successfully treated.

Don't say, "Life is unfair." Say, "Thank heaven I have the power to fix my problem."

Then get on with it.

Don't Compare Yourself to Others

This is a cardinal rule for dieters. Instead of wasting time on how others are doing with their fitness, concentrate on making yourself the best possible you.

Your need for reeducation in this area is vital.

What others do about their weight problems is up to them.

Focus on what *you* must do. Don't let thoughts of others interfere with your progress.

Make an Investment in Positive Thinking

To reinforce your newly developed positive actions and thoughts, read any of the excellent books available on the subject. Refer to the bibliography for some recommendations.

The more time and effort you invest in your reeducation, the more successful at weight maintenance you will be.

4. Images and Sensations

Imagery is a powerful tool.

If you've had emotional responses to vivid dreams, engrossing books, memories, daydreams, or fantasies, you already know the impact mental pictures can have.

When you learn how to use creative imagery to your advantage, you will have another tool to use against impulsive eating.

Here is a simple yet powerful bit of imagery that will enhance your positive thinking:

Picture yourself slender.

Be realistic, not perfectionistic. It's not helpful to visualize yourself as Bo Derek or Mr. America. Remember, perfectionism is negative.

In your mind's eye, see yourself from the front, back, and sides. Imagine what a lean you would look like.

Picture yourself in new clothing.

Visualize yourself in various situations and try to imagine the good feelings.

Begin to pair these images with everyday actions, such as getting dressed, taking a shower, brushing your teeth, and so on. In other words, each time you brush your teeth, create the image of yourself as a slender person. Soon the thoughts will appear automatically.

You are *not* conning yourself. You are working toward a very real goal as surely as if you were striving for a degree or a promotion.

You can use creative imagery in different ways to help your weight-loss program. For example, adverse mental imagery can be used to turn off some of the sensations associated with food.

Everybody has had the experience of being repulsed by food that was contaminated in some way. You can learn to evoke that appetite suppressant at will by practicing adverse creative imagery.

- Picture a long hair in your food
- Imagine unhealthful ingredients in the food
- Imagine that the food is dirty or contaminated
- Picture the food as globs of fat
- Imagine an eggshell in your food
- Picture the food doused with cold water or grease
- Picture yourself gaining weight with each bite

To see how effective this tool can be, use a scale of 1 to 10. Rate the food before you practice creative imagery and then rate it afterward. Test your ability to change the appeal of the food at will.

Decide ahead of time what kind of adverse imagery to use when you think you might be tempted with something you don't want to eat. Being prepared can help you avoid mistakes.

The technique of using adverse imagery is not designed to make eating a horrible experience. It is merely a practical, effective way of reducing your desire for junk food.

On the other hand, *positive* imagery can enhance your desire for more healthful foods.

When you eat lean meats, poultry, fish, and fresh fruits and vegetables, see yourself becoming slender.

Imagine that the food is making you healthier and stronger. In this way, foods that are slenderizing can become much more enjoyable.

Another way to counteract sensations that make you want to eat is to rechannel your thoughts. Rather than focus on the tempting food, think about something else that is pleasurable—music, art, conversation, et cetera.

Avoid daydreaming about food. Don't torture yourself with food magazines or cookbooks. Avoid watching cooking demonstrations on television. This goes for food commercials, too. Simply get up and leave the room.

Don't indulge in food fantasies (thoughts can lead to binging). Instead, write a letter, read a book, take a sauna, exercise, try a new hairstyle, or write your thoughts and feelings in your Snowbird Workbook.

5. Others

What do others have to do with your weight-loss commitment?
Plenty.

There will be people who will influence you one way or the other. And the best way to avoid bad influence and maximize encouragement is to become aware.

You will be encountering three types of people: the True Friend, the Police Officer, and the Saboteur.

The True Friend

This is a wonderful person to have in your corner. The True Friend wants what is best for you and attempts to help you achieve success every way he or she can.

Research studies have shown that support from an individual such as this can be an invaluable asset to the dieter.

The True Friend doesn't cajole, push, or nag.

The True Friend is positive and takes every opportunity to reinforce your smallest success.

The True Friend treats you as a dignified adult who has the right to make mistakes and the ability to achieve your goals.

If there is no True Friend in your life, it's worth cultivating one.

The Police Officer

These people usually mean well, but their methods are totally counterproductive.

They often monitor your eating. They try to order for you in restaurants. They'll take food out of your hands and off your plate. They like to give advice. They scrutinize your behavior and question your weight loss.

You'll recognize the Police Officers because their actions make you feel like a child caught with his hand in the cookie jar.

You experience guilt, humiliation, and, worst of all, resentment. While you may play "perfect" in their presence, behind their back you may feel the urge to eat twice as much.

It's very important to be assertive with these people. Tell them that you are capable of making your own decisions and mistakes.

If you have trouble being assertive, read any of the many good books on the subject (see the bibliography).

Many people who are overweight have difficulty with assertiveness. I often suggest taking an assertiveness-training course. Being assertive can go a long way in helping you achieve your goals.

The Saboteur

The Saboteur is a person who brings you fattening food knowing full well you are on a diet.

The Saboteur pushes food at you and then acts hurt or angry if you refuse.

You can spot the Saboteur by phrases such as:

"One little bite won't hurt."

"You can diet again tomorrow."

"I spent all day making this because I know it's your favorite."

"I'm so tired of your diet."

"You're no fun anymore."

"You look older when you lose weight."

"I think you're getting too skinny."

Et cetera.

The Saboteur behaves like a child who wants you to play his game.

Once again, the best way to deal with the Saboteur is to be assertive.

You need to be strong, hold your ground, and recognize that the Saboteur's motives are to derail your efforts.

Finally, it's important to recognize the True Friend, the Police Officer, and the Saboteur in yourself. If you are loving, understanding, and kind to yourself, it will be far easier to develop a positive outlook, motivation, and self-esteem.

On the other hand, if you police your actions, it will foster guilt, frustration, and binge eating.

If you act like the Saboteur, you will rationalize inappropriate eating habits, which will lead to discouragement and lack of motivation.

6. Fitness Forever!

Now that you've got the ball rolling, don't stop!

These techniques are not meant to be a temporary fix-it kit. They are designed to be incorporated into your thoughts and actions for a lifetime.

They will continue to open doors to self-awareness, compassion, understanding, and self-motivation. Their effects will spill over into other areas, permanently enhancing the quality of your life.

You need never suffer from eating problems again. You now have the tools to make winning changes.

Once you master FAT IS OFF! you can use it to unlearn the thoughts and actions that made you overweight in the first place.

Feelings. (Monitor and decode your urges to eat.)

Actions. (Take positive actions to change negative feelings.)

Thoughts. (Develop positive thinking.)

Images and *Sensations.* (Learn how to use creative imagery to control impulsive responses to food.)

Others. (Be aware that others can be a help or a hindrance.)

Fitness Forever! (Incorporate FAT IS OFF! into your life for good.)

Making Your Snowbird Workbook Work for You

The lists you have started in your workbook are there to help you avoid eating mistakes at a moment's notice.

Keep the workbook with you.

Add to it and read it regularly. Review positive thoughts and actions before you go to sleep and at quiet times throughout the day.

Whenever you feel the urge to eat, refer to your *Alternative Actions* list **before** you take a bite.

Even keeping a daily diary of your thoughts and successes can be a great help.

In short, *anything* that can help you achieve your goal of a slender lifetime can and should be kept in your Snowbird Workbook.

Review of Assignments for the Snowbird Workbook

1. Monitor your urges to splurge. Decode cravings for food and find out what feelings are behind them.

2. Make an *Alternative Actions* list to help you avoid eating during an appetite attack.

3. Make a list called *Why I Want to Lose Weight.*

4. Make a list called *Rewards for Good Behavior.*

5. Make a list called *Old Habits I Will Change* and begin to work on them one at a time.

6. Make a list called *Positive Thoughts for the Day.* Add a new thought each day and include compliments and words of encouragement you receive from others.

Examples of Alternative Actions

Take a bubble bath
Listen to a favorite tape or record
Buy a rose
Look through a gift catalogue (not food!)
Talk with a friend
Sing, play the piano, learn to play a recorder
Build something
Play golf or racquetball
Knit, needlepoint, or paint
Meditate
Have a manicure, pedicure, massage, or facial
Drink a large glass of sparkling water with a lime
Keep fresh vegetables clean and ready to eat in an appealing container
    in the fridge
Clean out the closet
Look through your photo albums
Take Spanish lessons
Take a long leisurely walk

Examples of Why I Want to Lose Weight

1. I'll enjoy feeling good
2. I love size 10!
3. Happiness is looking down and seeing the floor
4. I want to have more energy so I can spend more time with the kids and maybe take up tap dancing or skydiving!

5. I want to look more attractive
6. I'll plan that vacation that I wouldn't while I was heavy
7. I want people to look at me and think "wow"
8. I want to look 10 years younger
9. I want to look great at my high school reunion

Examples of Rewards for Good Behavior

1. Get a massage
2. Take a trip
3. Go to a concert
4. Buy new golf clubs, tennis racquet
5. Buy new furniture
6. Buy some new accessories (scarf, beads, tie, belt)
7. Buy a new swimsuit
8. Take tennis lessons

Examples of Old Habits I Will Change

1. Stop eating in bedroom and car
2. Cut down on sugar; eat more protein and complex carbohydrates
3. Stop eating while I'm talking on the phone
4. Be nice to myself with lots of things *other* than food
5. Stop putting myself down
6. Stop letting others make decisions about eating for me
7. Quit grocery shopping when I'm tired, bored, and hungry
8. Stop going without breakfast
9. Stop eating dinner late in the evening
10. Stop standing up and eating

Examples of Positive Thoughts for the Day

1. "I like myself, I don't need to be perfect"
2. "Every day I improve"
3. "I'm going to keep at it for as long as it takes"
4. "Just one step at a time"

5. "I love my ability to be sensitive, caring, realistic, compassionate, fun, interesting, etc."
6. "Jean loves the way I look in blue"
7. "I like the responsibility of taking control of my life and eating habits"
8. "I have a new haircut, I'm wearing a new dress, and I look great"
9. "I look better than I've looked in years"
10. "I deserve the best"

PART IV

The Keys to
a Slender Lifetime
or
Nothing Tastes as Good
as This Feels

10

The Snowbird Maintenance Plan

It's shocking but true. Over 95 percent of all dieters either fail to lose weight or are unable to maintain weight loss.

From that we can conclude that the blame should be placed squarely on the shoulders of the *diet*. Most diets were designed to fail.

There are many reasons why diets don't work. Most of them were discussed in chapter 1.

But the bottom line in many cases is this: *Most diets fail because they don't offer an effective, comprehensive, long-range maintenance plan.* Without such a maintenance plan there's no way a diet can ultimately succeed.

The Snowbird Maintenance Plan is simple, thorough, and effective. It works in conjunction with the other Snowbird components to help you achieve lasting weight control.

The Snowbird Maintenance Plan is designed to succeed. It is based on safe, proven strategies that focus on one point: vigorous maintenance is the most important element in lasting weight control.

The Snowbird Maintenance Plan can be likened to a three-legged stool. Each leg represents a different, but equally crucial component:

1. Regular exercise
2. Psychological awareness
3. Personal Eating Plan (PEP)

If any leg of the maintenance plan is missing, the program will not work. All three are equally vital for success.

How the Snowbird *Personal Eating Plan* Works

The Personal Eating Plan—or PEP—is designed to work not for just a few weeks but for an entire lifetime.

That's because overweight is a chronic metabolic disease that cannot be *cured*. But it can be successfully *treated*. Snowbird PEP is a lifetime treatment program.

Snowbird PEP is nutritionally balanced. It was designed to promote ongoing health and well-being. People can't live on a diet that leaves them tired, worn down, or nutritionally deficient.

Snowbird PEP is personalized. The plan works well because it treats each person as an individual. It teaches you to develop a lasting program based on your personal likes and dislikes.

Snowbird PEP is positive. Instead of dealing with negatives— "don't eat this and don't eat that"—it offers you an unlimited assortment of **dos.** This is a *lifetime* program. We don't want you to feel deprived in any way.

Snowbird PEP is realistic. You are not expected to go the rest of your life without socializing, dining out, entertaining, enjoying a cocktail, or eating your favorite foods. So we've found ways for you to include these things in your PEP without guilt or weight gain.

Snowbird PEP is simple. You don't have to count calories or eat the same foods day in and day out. The monotony and drudgery of other diets have been eliminated.

Snowbird PEP is flexible. Each person is unique. Therefore, Snowbird PEP doesn't try to squeeze you into a strict routine with no choices or variety. On the contrary, it encourages variety, excitement, interest, and constant change.

Snowbird PEP is convenient. It adjusts to your lifestyle—not the other way around. You can travel, enjoy good restaurants, and go to parties without going off your Personal Eating Plan. The Snowbird Maintenance Plan is truly a plan you can *live* with.

This is not to say that the Snowbird PEP does not require effort on your part. It certainly does.

It requires commitment, discipline, and perseverance but this is a small price to pay for a lifetime of slenderness and good health.

At the Southwest Bariatric Nutrition Center we spend many hours teaching and counseling each patient. We have found that the more support and knowledge the patients have about maintenance, the more successful they are.

That's why at the back of this book you will find a number of helpful books listed in the bibliography. Each one will offer insight, experience, encouragement, and knowledge to help you achieve your goal. The more you read, the more successful you are likely to be.

Together with your own Snowbird Workbook, you can strengthen, balance, and reinforce the three-legged stool called Maintenance.

Your Very Own *Personal Eating Plan*

Each *Personal Eating Plan*, or PEP, is composed of two distinct parts. One is called Basic PEP; the other is called Bonus PEP.

Basic PEP

Basic PEP is made up of a precise number of servings from six different food groups. Even though Basic PEP allows a wide variety of choices within each food group, it remains structured. This structure is necessary. It is the blueprint you will use to build a stable, nutritious maintenance program.

Basic PEP also ensures that caloric intake will be correct without your having to count calories. Protein, carbohydrate, and fat intake are balanced as well to prevent erratic swings in blood-insulin levels.

When Basic PEP is used exactly as prescribed, maintenance is virtually foolproof.

Bonus PEP

Bonus PEP ensures that maintenance will be satisfying and ultimately successful.

Why Is Bonus PEP So Important?

There are a number of reasons why Bonus PEP is so necessary to the Snowbird Maintenance Plan:

1. Bonus PEP Lets You Enjoy Special Treats

Many patients have said, "I can give up anything for a while, but I can't face the idea of *never* having my favorite food again."

All people have certain foods they cherish. Any maintenance plan that ignores this fact is going to fail.

After all, you are not moving to Mars. Sooner or later you will encounter one of your weaknesses and you will eat it, whether it's allowed or not.

Bonus PEP lets you have your special treats without forcing you to cheat or feel guilty.

Here's how it works. You are allowed a certain number of *Bonus* calories per day, which can be "spent" (like money) on anything you like. These calories can be spent each day, or saved up for something special. Naturally, the amount of calories in that special treat cannot exceed the *total* number of Bonus calories that have been saved.

Bonus calories are never high enough to allow uncontrolled eating binges to creep back into your life.

2. Bonus PEP Plans for "Hungry" Times

While Basic PEP gives you nutritious, filling meals and snacks, there are bound to be times when you will be hungrier than normal.

That's when Bonus PEP comes to the rescue.

Bonus calories can be used to have extras of any food. These Bonus calories are most wisely spent on wholesome, nutritious foods from any of the six food groups.

3. Bonus PEP Encourages You to Become Discriminating

Because Bonus calories are budgeted, patients learn to spend them on carefully chosen, highly satisfying, excellent-quality foods.

Very few patients decide to spend their precious Bonus calories on "empty" junk food.

4. Bonus PEP Lets You Have a Normal Social Life

By saving a few days' worth of Bonus calories, you can enjoy virtually any food served at a party or a restaurant.

Simply eat or drink whatever amount your Bonus calorie allowance will cover—and you can enjoy yourself free of guilt and extra pounds.

Remember: It's strictly *save now—spend later.* All Bonus calories *must* be saved in **advance**!

How to Make Bonus PEP Work

Eat Bonus calories in addition to, not instead of, your Basic PEP calories.

Look up the caloric value of the food you want to eat to determine how much of that food you may safely have.

Accumulate Bonus calories up to seven days in advance to cover the "cost" of high-calorie foods.

Eat your Bonus calories *only* in the weeks when your weight is within ideal weight range. (Ideal weight range is discussed later in this chapter.)

Eliminate all Bonus calories for the week if you are *above* your ideal weight range.

Add extra calories for the week if you are *below* your ideal weight range—100 calories per day for women and 150 for men.

Spend Bonus calories mostly on nutritious foods.

Plan ahead—Bonus calories must be premeditated.

Should You Take Vitamins?

The Snowbird *Personal Eating Plan*, while low in calories, is very high in nutrients. Still, I recommend that my patients supplement the Snowbird PEP with the same vitamins and minerals that are used in the Snowbird Diet.

In addition to your Snowbird PEP, you should take:

1. One Miles Laboratory 1-A-Day Vitamins with Minerals and Iron. *Do not* consume coffee or tea within 1 hour of taking the sup-

plement. Foods high in vitamin C (citrus fruits, broccoli, et cetera) will enhance the absorption of the iron from the supplement.

2. Calcium:* 1,000 mg. per day for men and premenopausal women; 1,500 mg. per day for postmenopausal women. Os-Cal is a good brand, but there are many others that are suitable. Do not take calcium if you have a problem with kidney stones. Calcium may be taken anytime, but most patients find that taking it at night enhances sleep.

What About Megavitamins?

Do not take any additional supplements. Many people have been conned into thinking megavitamins are necessary for good health.

They are not.

In fact, they may be dangerous to your health.

Here are some of the risks you invite when you take megadoses of vitamins:

- Extra supplements may be stored in the body in toxic (poisonous) amounts.
- Extra supplements may strain or exceed the capacity of the body's excretory system. When an excess of some vitamin is taken, the kidneys have to work harder to flush out the overload. (Because of the craze for megavitamins, it is said that Americans have the most expensive urine in the world!)
- By drastically increasing the intake of one vitamin or mineral, you may create a deficiency in another. Some nutrients taken in large quantities prevent the absorption of others. For example, too much zinc inhibits the absorption of copper. Too much vitamin C blocks the absorption of B_{12}. While this doesn't happen with nutrients from foods, it can occur with excessive vitamin-supplement intake.
- No supplement is guaranteed to be 100 percent nutritionally complete. Adequate protein, fiber, and trace minerals must be

---

*Research indicates that, whether dieting or not, unless a woman's diet is high in milk and cheese, after age 40 premenopausal women need a *daily* calcium intake of 1,000 mg, and postmenopausal 1,500 mg. for life, unless medically contraindicated. This will help prevent osteoporosis, or thin bones that break

supplied by food. Never take a megavitamin in place of eating a balanced meal.

In other words, megavitamins are a waste of money. Take only the vitamins recommended and you and your wallet will be a lot healthier.

You are now ready to learn how to put the Snowbird Maintenance Plan to work. The following pages include important charts, instructions, tips, hints, information, and reference material to help you achieve your goal of lasting weight management.

Our patients at the Southwest Bariatric Nutrition Center receive many hours of personal guidance and instruction on the subject. We have provided virtually the same guidance and instruction here.

Read it carefully. Refer to it often.

But most important, **put it to work.**

No diet can work if you don't use it.

I'm sure you've read *dos* and *don'ts* on other diets and probably ignored them.

Well, **now is the time to do it.**

The Snowbird Maintenance Plan works.

It will keep weight off permanently, but the diet can't do it alone. It needs a strong, determined partner—**you.**

THE SNOWBIRD PERSONAL EATING PLAN
A STEP-BY-STEP GUIDE

Step 1

The chart below is called the *Personal Eating Plan Blueprint.* When it is filled in, it will serve as a guide to help you plan daily maintenance menus.

Across the top are the six food groups: dairy (D); vegetable (V); fruit (FR); complex carbohydrates (CHO); protein (PR); fats and oils (F&O). At the back of this chapter you will find lists of foods in each of these six categories, for your convenience in planning menus.

To determine how many servings from each food group you will need per day, refer to the *Total Daily Servings Chart* on the following page.

PERSONAL EATING PLAN BLUEPRINT

Food Groups	D Dairy	V Vegetable	FR Fruits	CHO Complex Carbohydrates	PR Protein	F&O Fat & Oil
Total daily Servings						
Breakfast						
Lunch						
Dinner						
Snacks						

Bonus calories per day = _____

TOTAL DAILY SERVINGS

WOMEN	Group 1 D	Group 2 V	Group 3 FR	Group 4 CHO	Group 5 PR	Group 6 F&O
Age: Under 30	2	4+	3	4	10 oz.*	2
Age: 30–50	2	4+	3	3	9 oz.*	2
Age: Over 50	2	4+	2	3	8 oz.*	2

One alcoholic beverage per day is allowed on all plans

*Weight after cooking

MEN	Group 1 D	Group 2 V	Group 3 FR	Group 4 CHO	Group 5 PR	Group 6 F&O
Age: Under 30	2	4+	3	4	12 oz.*	3
Age: 30–50	2	4+	3	4	12 oz.*	2
Age: Over 50	2	4+	3	3	10 oz.*	2

One alcoholic beverage per day is allowed on all plans

*Weight after cooking

Write the *Total Daily Servings* for your sex and age in the correct spaces on the *Personal Eating Blueprint*.

Your *Total Daily Servings* **will not change** from day to day. They are fixed. Memorize them.

Step 2

The next step is to distribute the food throughout the day.

For guidance, refer to the *Suggested Distribution and Sample Menu*.

The sample menu is calculated for women under age 30. Variations on that menu for other sexes and ages follow.

Of course, the sample menus are merely a guide. You may distribute the food in any way that better suits you.

However, if you wish to vary the distribution of food, you should follow these rules:

1. Do include some food for breakfast.
2. Do include some protein at breakfast.
3. Do distribute food throughout the day rather than planning one huge meal in the evening.
4. Do allot some food for snacks, especially if you have a consistent "hungry" time of day.

SUGGESTED DISTRIBUTION
AND SAMPLE MENU
WOMEN UNDER 30

Food Category	D	V	FR	CHO	PR	F&O
Total daily Servings	2	4+	3	4	10	2
Breakfast	1	0	1	1	1 oz.	0
Lunch	0	2	0	1	3 oz.	1
Dinner	0	2	1	2	6 oz.	1
Snacks	1	0	1	0	0	0

Breakfast

¾ cup plain, low-fat yoghurt (1 D)

½ cup fresh blueberries (1 FR)

(Mix together, add calorie-free sweetener and a dash of allspice)

½ fork-split English muffin (1 CHO)

1 poached egg (1 ounce PR)

1 slice tomato, fresh basil (extra V)

(Toast muffin, top with egg, then tomato slice, sprinkle with
   pepper, salt [optional], and basil. Broil.)

Decaf coffee or tea

Lunch

GAZPACHO SOUP (1 V)

(Made with spicy tomato juice, any Group 2 vegetables, including diced carrot, cucumber, tomato, onion, celery, zucchini, plus Worcestershire, Tabasco, and/or herbs and seasonings to taste)

ORIENTAL PITA POCKET

½ whole-wheat pita (1 CHO)
Spread with tiny bit of hot Chinese mustard (free)
Stuff with 3 ounces tiny cooked shrimp (3 ounces PR) and shredded bok choy, bean sprouts, sliced mushrooms, and celery (1 V)
⅛ avocado (1 F&O)

Or:

CHICKEN PITA

Spread with regular mustard (free)
Stuff with 3 ounces sliced cold roast chicken (3 ounces PR) and sprouts, watercress, and mushrooms (1 V)
No-oil vinaigrette (free)
⅛ avocado (1 F&O)
Decaf cherry-almond tea (hot or cold)

Dinner

Fresh spinach salad (1 V) with 1 teaspoon oil in hot bacon dressing (1 F&O)
Ratatouille, stuffed (1 V)
Baked-potato half (1 CHO)
6 ounces grilled fresh salmon with green peppercorns and lemon (6 ounces PR)
1 glass Pinot Noir blanc
Decaf Swiss-blend coffee
Cinnamon/applesauce crepe (1 CHO) (1 FR)

Snack

1 small Bosc pear (1 FR)
1 ounce Camembert cheese (1 D)

WOMEN 30–50

Food Category	D	V	FR	CHO	PR	F&O
Total daily Servings	2	4+	3	3	9	2
Breakfast	1	0	1	1	1	0
Lunch	0	2	0	1	3	1
Dinner	0	2	1	1	5	1
Snacks	1	0	1	0	0	0

Menu

Same as women under 30 except:
Omit crepe at dinner; serve applesauce or baked apple
Decrease meat at dinner to 5 ounces

WOMEN OVER 50

Food Category	D	V	FR	CHO	PR	F&O
Total daily Servings	2	4+	2	3	8	2
Breakfast	1	0	1	1	1	0
Lunch	0	2	0	1	3	1
Dinner	0	2	1	1	4	1
Snacks	1	1	0	0	0	0

Menu

Same as women under 30 except:
Omit crepe at dinner; serve applesauce or baked apple
Decrease meat at dinner to 4 ounces
Omit fruit at snack; substitute raw vegetable

MEN UNDER 30

Food Category	D	V	FR	CHO	PR	F&O
Total Daily Servings	2	4+	3	4	12	3
Breakfast	1	0	1	1	2	0
Lunch	0	2	0	1	4	1
Dinner	0	2	1	2	6	2
Snacks	1	0	1	0	0	0

Menu

Same as women under 30 except:
Breakfast—add 1 ounce low-fat mozzarella cheese to egg
Lunch—increase meat to 4 ounces
Dinner—add 1 extra teaspoon of salad dressing

MEN 30–50

Food Category	D	V	FR	CHO	PR	F&O
Total daily Servings	2	4+	3	4	12	2
Breakfast	1	0	1	1	2	0
Lunch	0	2	0	1	4	1
Dinner	0	2	1	2	6	1
Snacks	1	0	1	0	0	0

Menu

Same as women under 30 except:
Breakfast—add 1 ounce low-fat mozzarella cheese to egg
Lunch—increase meat to 4 ounces

MEN OVER 50

Food Category	D	V	FR	CHO	PR	F&O
Total daily Servings	2	4+	3	3	10	2
Breakfast	1	0	1	1	1	0
Lunch	0	2	0	1	3	1
Dinner	0	2	1	1	6	1
Snacks	1	0	1	0	0	0

Menu

Same as women 30–50 except:
Dinner—protein serving is 6 ounces

If you write a food-distribution plan into the spaces remaining in the PEP Blueprint, you will have some idea of how your personal Blueprint will look.

You will always be working with the same number of daily servings from each of the six food groups. The only thing that will change might be your pattern of distribution.

It helps to memorize your Total Daily Servings.

Patients say that after three weeks, making up the Blueprint becomes as automatic as their old unhealthful eating pattern used to be.

It takes a little practice. But it's easy and *very* rewarding.

Use the PEP Blueprint format to draw your own Blueprints for each day. I recommend that patients keep their Blueprints in their own Snowbird Workbooks for easy reference.

Some patients prefer not to vary food distribution daily. They make one plan and stick to it each day. This is a bit simpler and less time-consuming, but if your schedule permits variation, by all means make up a different distribution plan as called for.

Assuming you stick to one distribution plan, here's what the Blueprint would tell you at a glance:

1. How many servings from each food group to have each day
2. When to eat
3. How many Bonus calories per day you are entitled to

Step 3

Next you will learn how to calculate your daily Bonus PEP, or free calories.

This chart tells precisely how many Bonus calories you are allowed per day.

WOMEN		MEN	
AGE: under 30	150	**AGE:** under 30	200
AGE: 30 to 50	100	**AGE:** 30 to 50	150
AGE: over 50	75	**AGE:** over 50	100

Enter the exact number of Bonus calories you are allowed each day into the space provided under the PEP Blueprint.

To determine the number of calories in the foods you wish to eat, consult a reliable calorie counter. Check the bibliography for recommendations.

Remember: Bonus calories must be saved *before* they can be spent. Don't have a fattening dessert tonight thinking you can save up your Bonus calories for the next two weeks. **That won't work.**

You must accumulate Bonus calories before you can use them.

If you wish to spend your Bonus calories by the day, that's fine. But if you want to eat something that has more calories than your daily allotment, you must save them up.

Step 4

The next step—and a very important one—is to keep a food diary.

Keeping a food diary is an absolute *must* during the first two months of the Snowbird Maintenance Plan.

Many patients find they like keeping a food diary so much that they continue to do so long after the first two months.

Keeping a food diary is important for many reasons.

For one thing, once your food plan is committed to paper you won't have to worry about it. Not being preoccupied with food is a blessing.

Another reason for keeping a food diary is that once your food plan is written down, you are less likely to make mistakes. If you forget what you are supposed to eat, simply refer to the written plan. This can eliminate momentary weaknesses and impulsive eating.

Carefully planning a menu on paper *before* you eat assures you of a balanced, nutritious diet. You won't eat haphazardly.

Keeping a food diary helps you establish good, new eating habits. You won't be as likely to backslide.

Finally, a food diary is a positive record of the investment you are making in your new way of life. You can refer to it whenever you need to. It will serve as a guide to and a reminder of your new positive approach to eating.

How to Keep a Food Diary

1. Use your Personal Eating Plan Blueprint for guidance in selecting foods and spacing them throughout the day.
2. Refer to the PEP Daily Diary on the following pages for guidance in creating your food diary.
3. It helps to write your Daily Food Diary in a section of your Snowbird Workbook for convenience and easy reference.
4. Vary your menus each day to reflect seasonal foods. *Do not use the same foods over and over.* This is not healthful and becomes very boring.
5. Keep careful, accurate records. Write down everything—all your foods and all your drinks.
6. Choose foods that fulfill the requirements of Basic PEP.

PEP DAILY FOOD DIARY

BASIC PEP	FOOD	GROUP	AMOUNT
Breakfast	_____	_____	_____
	_____	_____	_____
	_____	_____	_____
Lunch	_____	_____	_____
	_____	_____	_____
	_____	_____	_____
Dinner	_____	_____	_____
	_____	_____	_____
	_____	_____	_____
Snack	_____	_____	_____
	_____	_____	_____
	_____	_____	_____

BONUS PEP	FOOD EATEN	CALORIES
	_____	_____
	_____	_____
	_____	_____

BONUS PEP CALORIES SAVED TODAY _____

EXERCISE DONE TODAY

Type _____

Duration _____

Target Heart Rate _____

PEP DAILY FOOD DIARY

BASIC PEP	FOOD	GROUP	AMOUNT
Breakfast	Cantaloupe wedge	1 PR	¼
	Bagel with	1 CHO	½
	mozzarella cheese	1 D	1 oz.
	Scrambled egg	1 PR	1
Lunch	_Chef Salad_ { Salad greens, tomatoes, carrots, mushrooms,	2 V	unlimited
	Turkey and ham strips	3 PR	3 oz.
	crackers	1 CHO	8
	Italian dressing	1 F+O	2 tsp.
Dinner	Sliced tomatoes and cucumbers, bread strips	1 V / 1 CHO	unlimited
	Boiled shrimp	6 PR	6 oz
	Baked potato	1 CHO	1 small
	Butter	1 F+O	1 tsp.
	steamed broccoli	V	unlimited
	Baked pear	1 FR	1
Snack	Plain lowfat yoghurt with	D	¾ cup
	Strawberries and sweetened	FR	¾ cup

BONUS PEP	FOOD EATEN	CALORIES
	Sherbet ½ cup	130

BONUS PEP CALORIES SAVED TODAY _____ 20

EXERCISE DONE TODAY

Type _Swimming_

Duration _30 minutes_

Target Heart Rate _140_

THIS IS A SAMPLE DAY FOR A WOMAN UNDER 30.

7. Always include the Bonus PEP calories that were either saved or spent for the day. If you saved 75 calories, enter "+75." If you spent 75 calories, enter "−75." Keep a running total of *accumulated* Bonus calories from day to day.

8. Weigh and measure all food carefully to be absolutely sure of portions. This is to ensure that you don't *undereat.* Many patients tend to underestimate portions when they begin maintenance. Eat what is required on your Blueprint—no more, no less.

9. Enter your exercise plan for the day. Record the type of exercises you plan to do along with the duration and your target heart rate.

That's it. The first complete page in your Daily Food Diary. Soon it will become second nature. You are now well on your way to unlocking the door to a lifetime of slimness and good health.

What Is Ideal Weight Range?

Most people think their ideal weight is a static number—that it should never fluctuate.

This is a mistaken assumption.

Nobody can possibly weigh the same every single day, day in and day out.

Yet I hear patients say things like, "I want to weigh 142 pounds."

They don't realize that weighing 142 pounds consistently is *impossible.*

There are too many variables.

Body weight normally fluctuates as much as 3 to 6 pounds.

How much you weigh from day to day depends on several factors—fluid balance, fullness of the digestive tract and bladder, and hormonal states, to name a few.

Because of this constant, normal fluctuation of weight, it is sensible to think of your weight in terms of a *weight range,* rather than an unchanging number.

When you practice good maintenance habits, the focus should *not* be on the scale. Don't keep hopping on and off to see how you're doing.

If you do, your normal weight fluctuations are likely to lead you to undereat or overeat—and both are counterproductive to successful maintenance.

Instead, direct your attention and effort into planning the proper foods, exercising, and focusing on behavior improvements—*not* on weighing yourself each time you pass a scale.

If you cheat, don't run to the scale to see if you've gained any weight. Remember, it may not show up right away. In fact, it may not show up for quite a while. But eventually it *will* show up. **Nobody cheats and gets away with it.**

To maintain your weight, calories going in must be balanced by energy going out. When you take in more food than you need, the excess calories will invariably turn up as stored fat.

Determining Your Ideal Weight Range

At the Southwest Bariatric Nutrition Center, ideal weight ranges are determined by using a number of factors.

First we evaluate the patient's weight history.

We also consider the ease with which that patient is able to maintain certain weights.

We also do body composition analysis by computer. This is a new way to determine what percentage of the body is actually fat tissue. The computerized body composition analysis is a far more significant guide to total health than is actual body weight.

For example, a man who is 6 feet tall and weighs 200 pounds might have 18 percent body fat. He would be within his ideal weight range.

But another man of the same height and weight range might have 30 percent body fat, which would indicate that he is *overweight*. Remember also that your percentage of body fat usually increases with age.

Using computerized projections and other criteria, we can accurately pinpoint each person's ideal weight range. A qualified physician or nutritionist can help you do the same.

The following chart offers general guidelines to help you determine your ideal weight range without the help of a professional.

For men, the ideal body fat is between 12 percent and 20 percent. Anything over that is considered overweight.

In women, ideal body fat ranges from 18 percent to 25 percent.

Differences in natural body fat are one reason why men lose weight more quickly than women. They have naturally higher levels of lean body mass, or muscle. Muscle is active and demands more energy, thus using up more calories. Fat, on the other hand, is inert and demands nothing. It's easy to see, then, that a body with more lean muscle tissue will burn calories faster than a body with a high percentage of fat.

Because there is no accurate way to measure your percent of body fat, the Body Mass Index (BMI) is used to determine to what degree you are overweight and to find your ideal body weight. At the First International Meeting on Body Weight Control in Montreux, Switzerland, in April, 1985, it was explained that the BMI does *not* indicate your percent of body fat, but rather expresses your weight in kilos over your height in meters squared. Obesity is classified on page 000.

Weigh Yourself Properly

Again, I caution you not to jump on and off the scale each time you pass one. This is destructive to maintenance.

Instead, follow these simple tips, and the scale will never be your worst enemy.

- Weigh yourself no more than once a week.
- Always weigh yourself at the same time under the same conditions. If possible, weigh yourself in the morning with an empty bladder, before you have anything to eat or drink. It's preferable to weigh yourself nude, but if you weigh yourself fully clothed, do it the same each week. Consistency is a must.
- If you weigh more than your ideal weight range, watch your food more closely. Weigh and measure everything. Keep careful records. Eliminate Bonus calories until you are back within your ideal range.

* BODY MASS INDEX

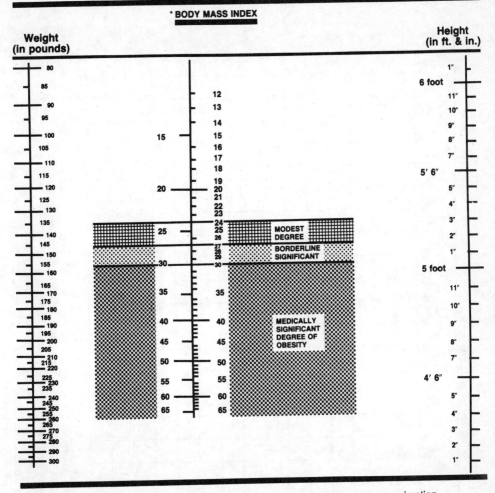

Weight (in pounds)

Height (in ft. & in.)

With a ruler draw a line from your height to your weight. This will give you an approximation of your BODY MASS INDEX in Kilogram/Meters^2

*Classification of Obesity using Body Mass Index:

Grade	BMI (Kg/M^2)**	Class
0	20–25	Normal
I	25–30	Moderate
II	30–40	Severe
III	40 plus	Very Severe

**Kilogram/Meters^2

Treatment using Body Mass Index:

BMI	Treatment
20–25	None
25–30	Treat especially if other risk factors are positive—i.e. High Blood Pressure, Diabetes, etc.
30–40	Treatment always necessary
40 plus	Treat vigorously and manditory

(Reference: Kays A, Fidanza F, Karvonen MJ, Kimura N, and Taylor HL:. Indices of Relative Weight and Obesity, J. Chronic Diseases 25:329, 1973).

WEEKLY WEIGH-IN

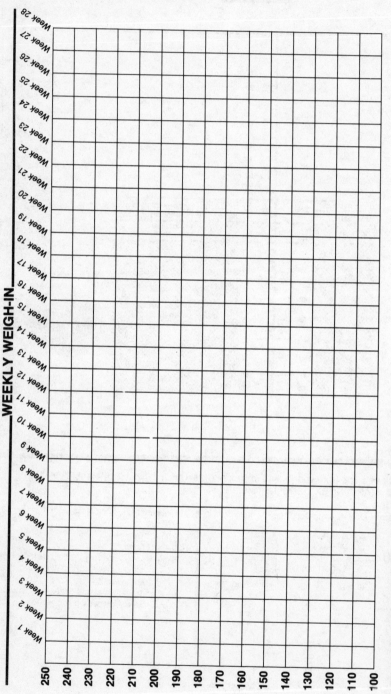

Week 1 Week 2 Week 3 Week 4 Week 5 Week 6 Week 7 Week 8 Week 9 Week 10 Week 11 Week 12 Week 13 Week 14 Week 15 Week 16 Week 17 Week 18 Week 19 Week 20 Week 21 Week 22 Week 23 Week 24 Week 25 Week 26 Week 27 Week 28

250 240 230 220 210 200 190 180 170 160 150 140 130 120 110 100

MAINTENANCE FINE-TUNING INSTRUCTIONS

1. Mark your ideal weight range by drawing a red line across the graph at the upper and lower weight numbers of your range.
2. Weigh yourself at the same day, same time, same conditions, same scale, once a week.
3. If your weekly weight falls within the **red lines**, continue with your successful food and exercise choices.
4. If your weight is *below* the bottom red line, add 100 Bonus calories for **women** and 150 Bonus calories for **men** to your *daily* total of Bonus calories.
5. If your weight is *above* the top red line, **omit all Bonus calories** for the week.

Personal Eating Plan Review

Here is a quick rundown of the elements in PEP:

1. The Basic portion of PEP provides a specific number of servings per day from each of the six food groups. Basic PEP is essential for good nutrition and should be followed carefully. Foods should be distributed throughout the day, not concentrated at one meal. All foods within a category are considered calorically equal.

2. The Bonus portion of PEP concerns extra calories that make maintenance work for you and your lifestyle. Bonus PEP is based on a specific allotment of calories per day. These calories may be used day by day or saved up to use on something more caloric. Bonus calories should not be saved longer than 7 days. Bonus PEP is to be used *only* when your weight falls within your ideal weight range.

3. Take only the supplements recommended in this book. Any other supplements should be taken under the care of a physician.

THE SIX FOOD GROUPS

The six food groups in your Personal Eating Plan are dairy, vegetables, fruits, complex carbohydrates, protein, and fats and oils.

Within a single group, all the foods are interchangeable. But you cannot trade a fruit for a vegetable, a vegetable for a protein, and so on.

The food-group lists included in this book are by no means complete. Rather, they are intended to include high-quality basic foods that will be the mainstay of your PEP.

If you wish to include foods not on these lists, you may use any of the exchange lists of the American Diabetes Association (see the bibliography). The servings in the Snowbird Maintenance Plan are also interchangeable with those on the American Diabetes Association exchange lists.

Group 1

Dairy

Dairy products are *essential* to your Personal Eating Plan.

Foods in this group supply vital protein, calcium, magnesium, and vitamins A and D.

Do not omit this group without consulting a physician or nutritionist.

- High-fat dairy products such as cream, cream cheese, and butter are listed in Group 6—fats and oils.
- Frozen dairy products such as ice cream, ice milk, and frozen yoghurt must come from *Bonus calories*.
- The only difference between nonfat and whole or 2-percent dairy products is the fat content. If you choose to use whole or 2-percent products, instead of *skim* or nonfat products, they should be counted as both Group 1—dairy, *and* Group 6—fats and oils (see list).
- The cheeses listed may be counted as *either* Group 1—dairy, or Group 5—protein.
- Each food is listed below in the amount equal to *one serving*.

MILK PRODUCTS

Skim or nonfat milk	8 oz. (1 cup)
Powdered nonfat dry milk	⅓ cup (powder)
Canned evaporated skim milk	½ cup
Buttermilk made from skim milk	1 cup
Plain low-fat yoghurt	¾ cup

CHEESES

Brie	1 oz.
Camembert	1 oz.
Cottage, low-fat	⅓ cup
Edam	1 oz.
Feta	1 oz.
Liederkranz	1 oz.
Limburger	1 oz.
Mozzarella, part skim	1 oz.
Mysost	1 oz.

Port du Salut	1 oz.
Provolone	1 oz.
Ricotta, part skim	¼ cup
Tilsit	1 oz.
Tivoli Danalette	1 oz.

Count the following as 1 dairy *and* 1 fat serving:

2-percent milk	8 oz. (1 cup)
Canned evaporated low-fat milk	½ cup

Count the following as 1 dairy *and* 2 fat servings:

Whole milk	8 oz. (1 cup)
Buttermilk made from whole milk	8 oz. (1 cup)
Canned evaporated whole milk	½ cup

Group 2

Vegetables

The vegetables in this group are nutritional wonders. They're miraculously low in calories, yet they supply an abundance of crucial vitamins, minerals, and whole fiber.

Whole fiber is essential to dieters for many reasons. One of its best qualities is that it gives a feeling of comfortable fullness without adding too many calories. Any dieter knows it's a lot easier to stick to a diet when his or her stomach isn't grumbling for food.

- Vegetables in this group may be eaten raw or cooked in *any amount desired*. Years of research at the Southwest Bariatric Nutrition Center show that you get full before you get fat!
- The letters A and C after a vegetable indicate that it is a good source of vitamins A and/or C.
- Always include one source of vitamin C per day, either vegetable or fruit.

- For ideas to enhance the flavors of these vegetables, refer to *Unlimited Foods.*
- Starchy vegetables such as peas, dried beans, legumes, potatoes, squash, and corn are listed in Group 4—complex carbohydrates.
- High-fat items such as avocados and olives are listed in Group 6—fats and oils.

Anise or fennel (A)
Artichoke (A)
Asparagus (A,C)
Beans—green, wax, snap, sprouts
Beets
Bok choy—(Chinese greens) (A)
Broccoli (A,C)
Brussels sprouts (A,C)
Cabbage—red, Napa, savoy (C)
Carrots (A)
Cauliflower (C)
Celeriac (celery root)
Celery
Chicory (A)
Cilantro (Chinese parsley)
Cucumber
Daikon (white radish) (C)
Eggplant
Endive
Escarole (A)
Ginger root
Green pepper (A,C)
Greens, all types (A,C)—
mustard greens, dandelion greens, chicory, beet tops, etc.
Herbs
Jicama (Mexican root)
Leeks

Lettuce
Mushrooms—Asian, dried, enoki, any type
Okra
Onions
Oyster plant
Parsley
Pea pods—Oriental peas, snow peas
Peppers—green, red, chile (A,C)
Pickles, not sweet
Radishes
Rutabaga (C)
Sauerkraut
Shallots
Sorrel
Spinach (A,C)
Sprouts (C)
Squash, summer types— crookneck, pattypan, yellow
Swiss chard (A,C)
Tomatillos (A,C)
Tomatoes (A,C)
Tomato juice (A,C)*
Turnips (C)
Vegetable juice cocktail (A,C)*
Water chestnuts
Watercress (A,C)
Zucchini

*Do not use more than 1 cup per day

Group 3

Fruits

Like vegetables, fruits are rich in vitamins, minerals, and fiber. But since they are higher in natural sugar (and therefore calories), fewer and smaller servings are recommended.

It's best to eat fruit raw and, if possible, unpeeled. For one thing, it's more filling. It also has more fiber and nutrition than processed fruit or fruit juice.

Whenever there's a choice between whole, raw fruit and juice, choose the fruit. Fruit juice should be consumed infrequently because it is higher in calories and lower in fiber than raw fruit. It's also less filling.

Never drink fruit juice with added sugar or syrup.

- The letters A and C after a fruit indicate that it is a good source of vitamins A and/or C.
- Always include one source of vitamin C per day, either fruit or vegetable.
- Each food is listed in the amount equal to *one serving*.

Apple	1 small or ½ large
Apple juice	⅓ cup
Applesauce	½ cup
Apricots, fresh or dried (A)	2 (4 halves)
Avocado	See *Fats*
Banana	½
Blueberries	½ cup
Blackberries	½ cup
Cantaloupe (A,C)	¼ of 6″ diameter melon
Carambola	3 ½ oz.
Casaba melon (C)	1 cup
Cherimoya (tropical fruit)	1 ¾ oz.
Cherries	10
Cider	⅓ cup
Cranberries (unsweetened)	Unlimited
Cranshaw melon	2″ wedge
Dates	2
Figs	1

Fruit cocktail	½ cup
Gooseberries (C)	⅔ cup
Grapefruit (C)	½
Grapefruit juice (C)	½ cup
Grapes	12
Grape juice	¼ cup
Guava (C)	⅔
Honeydew melon (C)	⅛
Kiwi (C)	1 large
Kumquats (C)	2 small
Lemon (C)	1 large
Lime (C)	2
Loganberries	⅔ cup
Mandarin orange (C)	½ cup
Mango (A,C)	1
Nectar, any type	¼ cup
Nectarine (A)	1 small
Orange (C)	1
Orange juice (C)	½ cup
Papaya (A,C)	¾ cup
Peach (A)	1 small
Pear	1 small
Persimmon (A)	½ large
Pineapple	½ cup
Pineapple juice	⅓ cup
Plums	2
Pomegranate	1
Prickly pear	3 oz.
Prunes	2
Prune juice	¼ cup
Raisins	2 T.
Raspberries (C)	½ cup
Strawberries (C)	¾ cup
Tangelo (C)	1
Tangerine	1
Watermelon (C)	(C) ¾ cup

Group 4

Complex Carbohydrates

Everyone knows that bread and potatoes are fattening. Right?

Wrong!

Complex carbohydrates, including breads, potatoes, and other high-quality starches, are *not* high in calories.

The key to enjoying these foods without gaining weight is to limit the size and number of servings.

Complex carbohydrates often are ideal sources of B vitamins, iron, and fiber. To get the most nutritional value from this group, choose mostly whole-grain products.

Whole-grain products are often labeled "whole wheat," "unrefined," "bran," or any other phrase that indicates that the entire grain kernel—whether wheat, oat, corn, rice, et cetera—has been used. Whole-grain products contain more fiber and trace minerals than do their refined, enriched counterparts.

- Bread: It is difficult to judge serving sizes for the various types of breads. If the package contains a nutrition label, have the amount or size slice that is equal to 1 oz. If home baked or bakery bread is used, visualize a serving size equal to 1 slice of average (albeit tasteless) sandwich bread.
- Each food is listed in the amount equal to *one serving*.

BREAD

Bread, any type	1 slice or equivalent
Bagel, plain	½
Breadsticks, 9"	3 average, ⅔ oz.
Crepe (pancake only)	1 large
Cornbread	1 cube, 1½"
Dinner roll	1 small
English muffin	½
Pita bread	½ large
Tortilla, corn or flour	1 6" round
Melba toast	6

CEREALS

Natural cold cereals (unsweetened), dry	¾ cup
Cooked cereal	½ cup

GRAIN PRODUCTS AND OTHER STARCHES

Barley, cooked	½ cup
Cornmeal, cooked or raw	2 T.
Cornstarch	2 T.
Flour	2½ T.
Rice, cooked	½ cup
Pasta, any type, cooked	½ cup
Wheat germ	2 T.
Wild rice, cooked	½ cup

CRACKERS AND SNACKS

Graham crackers	2 squares
Lahvosh	1 medium
Matzoh	½ large
Popcorn, no oil used in popping	3 cups
Pretzels, thin stick	20
Pretzels, 3-ring	5
Rice crackers	6
Snack crackers (Wheat Thins, Triscuits, etc.)	8 (avoid high-fat types)
Soda crackers	5 squares
Water crackers	4 small or 2 large

STARCHY VEGETABLES

Beans, starchy—pinto, navy, black, cannellini, etc.	½ cup
Black-eyed peas	½ cup
Corn	⅓ cup or ½ ear
Garbanzo beans	⅓ cup
Hominy	½ cup
Lentils	⅓ cup
Lima beans	⅓ cup
Parsnips	⅔ cup
Peas, all types	½ cup
Potato, sweet	¼ cup
Potato, red, new, white	½ cup
Pumpkin	¾ cup
Squash, winter, acorn	½ cup
Yams	¼ cup

Group 5

Protein

Although many foods contain protein, only the foods in this list (and some in Group 1) are complete *body-building* proteins.

Protein-rich foods are excellent sources of B vitamins as well as iron and zinc.

To find out how much of these foods you should have each day, refer to the Personal Eating Plan. It will list your daily protein portion in ounces. Food should be weighed *after* cooking. Do not include the weight of bones.

- All visible fat should be removed before cooking.
- Poultry should be eaten without skin.
- Raw meat will weigh ¼ to ⅓ less after cooking. Fish will weigh ⅕ less. Buy enough to ensure the right amount *after* cooking.
- Weigh each portion carefully on an accurate kitchen scale. This is to make sure you are giving yourself large enough portions. Many people mistakenly think the servings are smaller than they really are. Continue to weigh all servings until you can accurately judge portions at a glance.
- Use cooking methods that add few or no calories. Baking, roasting, microwaving, broiling on a rack, steaming, poaching, and grilling are good choices.
- Meats that are stewed or boiled should be cooled completely so congealed fat can easily be skimmed off the top.
- Protein foods are listed here in three categories, divided according to their fat content.

Remember to refer to the Personal Eating Plan to determine serving sizes.

Lean Proteins

BEEF
Very lean baby beef
Very lean ground round
Lean chuck
Flank steak
Tenderloin
Top and bottom round
Rump

FISH
All types, fresh or frozen
Canned in water or brine
All shellfish, fresh, frozen, or canned, water or brine
Sardines, without oil

GAME MEATS
Buffalo
Venison
Quail
Squab
Rabbit

LAMB
Leg and shoulder cuts
Rib
Sirloin
Shank

PORK
Ham, extra lean
Leg
Rump
Smoked center slices

POULTRY (eaten without skin)
Chicken
Cornish hen
Ground turkey
Guinea hen
Pheasant
Turkey

VEAL
Leg
Loin
Shank
Shoulder

NON-MEAT PROTEIN
Tofu, 3½ oz. equals 1 oz. protein

Medium-Fat Proteins

Limit these to four servings per week or less.

BEEF
Chuck
Corned beef, fresh or canned
Lean ground
Rib eye
Sirloin

LAMB
Chops

PORK
Boston butt
Canadian bacon
Chops
Ham, boiled
Ham, picnic
Loin
Shoulder cuts

POULTRY
Turkey sausage
Turkey cold cuts

ORGAN MEATS
Heart
Kidney
Liver
Sweetbreads

VEAL
Cutlets

CHEESE, PART SKIM
Brie
Camembert
Cottage cheese, low-fat — ¼
cup equals 1 oz. protein
Edam
Feta or Chèvre (goat cheese)
Limburger
Mozzarella, part skim
Mysost
Pot cheese
Ricotta, part skim
Tilsit

EGGS
1 egg equals 1 oz. protein

High-Fat Proteins

Because of the high fat content, these foods should not be eaten often—never more than 1 serving per week.

BEEF
Brisket
Hamburger
Prime rib
Steaks—rib, club, T-bone

LAMB
Breast

PORK
Back ribs
Country ham
Ground
Sausage
Spare ribs

POULTRY
Capon
Duck
Goose

VEAL
Breast

CHEESE
All types not listed under
    medium-fat proteins, except
    cream cheese

PEANUT BUTTER
2 T. equals 1 oz. meat plus 1
    serving fat

Group 6

Fats and Oils

Fats are not unhealthy *when used sparingly*. They should not be eliminated from a healthful diet. In fact, in very small amounts they are beneficial.

When they are added to food, fats make a dish more flavorful and satisfying.

But remember, fats are highly concentrated with calories.

If you use even a little bit more than you should, you may find yourself inching back up the scale.

Learn to enjoy their delicate flavors in small, sensible amounts and you can eat them without guilt—and without gaining.

Don't eliminate them—but don't overdo them either.

- Each food is listed in the amount equal to *one serving.*

Avocado	1 slice (⅛ whole)
Bacon	1 slice
Bacon fat	1 tsp.
Butter	1 tsp.
Cream, heavy	2 tsp.
Cream, half and half	1 T.
Cream cheese	1 T.
Hollandaise	1 T.
Margarine	1 tsp.
Mayonnaise	1 tsp.
Olives	5
Oil, any type	1 tsp.
Salad dressing, homemade 1 part oil to 1 part vinegar	2 tsp.
Salt pork	1″ cube
Sour cream	½ T.
Tartar sauce	½ T.
White sauce, medium	2 T.

NUTS AND SEEDS

Almonds	10
Brazils	2
Cashews	6
Macadamias	3
Pecans	2
Spanish peanuts	2
Regular peanuts	10
Pistachios	20
Seeds	2 tsp.
Walnuts	6

Unlimited Foods

These foods have so few calories they can be considered calorie-free when eaten in normal amounts. Be sure to put these foods at the top of your shopping list.

Unlimited Foods

These foods have so few calories they can be considered calorie-free when eaten in normal amounts. Be sure to put these foods at the top of your shopping list.

Decaf coffee, tea, diet soda
Sparkling waters (except tonic
    water and collins mix, which
    have high sugar content)
Calorie-free beverage mixes
Fat-free broth and bouillon
    cubes
Dry cocoa powder—limit to
    1 T. daily
Herbs, fresh or dried
Spices
Flavor extracts

Low-calorie and unflavored
    gelatins
Mustard
Horseradish
Soy sauce
Worcestershire
Salts, all types
Pepper
Vinegar
Pan-coating sprays
Salad dressings with fewer than
    10 calories per serving

11

Living the Snowbird Lifestyle
Dining Out, Traveling, and
Entertaining Without Gaining Weight

Congratulations. You've done it. You and the Snowbird Diet
are a winning combination!
    You've discovered that losing weight is not as difficult as
it once may have seemed.

You have made a personal commitment to a lifetime of being
slender.

You have climbed the mountain.

But, as any experienced mountain climber will tell you, there are
just as many perils on the way down as there were going up.

From now on, you will be living strictly in the real world. You will
be making your way on your own.

There are bound to be stumbling blocks.

Be prepared for them.

Remember that overweight is a chronic problem that cannot be
cured—it can only be *treated*. The treatment, from now on, is in your
hands.

Because of the Snowbird Diet, you are better prepared now than
at any other time in your life. You are slender. You are strong and fit.
You have a better understanding of what made you overweight. You
are armed with insight and information.

The Snowbird Maintenance Plan has illuminated your path to a
future of fitness and wellness.

If you practice maintenance enthusiastically, *you will never be fat again.*

But don't make the mistake of thinking that maintenance will be a breeze.

It requires constant vigilance.

There are many pitfalls—pushy waiters, "friendly" saboteurs, well-meaning relatives, people who are envious of your new image, to name just a few.

But remember: For every fattening problem there is a slender solution.

Focus on these slender solutions. Arm yourself with determination. You *will* succeed.

You have made a great investment in yourself. You have done something for yourself that no one could have done for you. You have learned to respect your body and your health. You have learned to love yourself. You now know what it is to be the best possible you.

You are finally the successful person you were always meant to be.

Bear that in mind as you face the fattening foibles of the real world.

Snowbird's Slender Solutions

This chapter is filled with words of wisdom on maintaining your weight loss. None of them will work if you don't use them.

They are to be taken seriously.

Remember that most dieters fail in maintenance.

The temptations that made you fat before are still lurking out there.

You must learn how to handle them in ways that are positive and healthful.

Mental Imagery in Maintenance

As you read this chapter, make notes on the Slender Solutions that particularly apply to your life.

Mentally incorporate them into your repertoire of reactions.

For instance, if you have trouble ordering the proper foods when faced with a tempting menu, begin to imagine yourself in that very situation.

Picture yourself ordering the correct food.

Picture the waiter.

Imagine yourself being assertive. Tell him in no uncertain terms what you want and how you would like it prepared.

Imagine sending it back if it isn't right—all the time being friendly, but firm.

Practice this mental imagery whenever you can—in the shower, on your way to work, at night before you go to bed. You'll be amazed how powerful a tool this is.

When you are faced with the real situation, you will have rehearsed it mentally to the point where proper actions come almost as second nature.

This kind of positive mental imagery works for any situation that you presently feel ill at ease with or insecure about.

It's a positive-thinking tool that has been successful for many people.

While positive mental imagery pays off, there is no substitute for the confidence building that comes when you master situations that once were your downfall.

Practice taking control of situations one at a time. Don't try to do so much that you are overwhelmed.

Be steady, persevering, and patient.

Before you know it, you'll wonder how these "problems" ever got the best of you.

From now on, you control food—it does not control you.

Slender Solutions:
The Snowbird Dines Out

On the average, Americans eat out at least once a day. Most Snowbirds exceed that average.

This means that learning how to handle life at a restaurant table is crucial.

Can't decide what to order? Afraid you'll blow it? Is the waiter intimidating?

Here are Snowbird's Slender Solutions:

- Develop the attitude that dining out is a natural part of your life. It is **not** a special event that might give you an excuse to overeat.
- Choose a restaurant that offers a variety of foods that can be prepared to your specifications. In other words, don't decide to go to a place that serves only the things you should not eat. You'd be surprised how many gourmet restaurants prepare special light meals. The internationally known Four Seasons restaurant in New York is becoming as well known for its "Spa" cuisine as its gourmet food. Call ahead for details.
- Avoid fast-food restaurants. Their choices are usually extremely limited and they emphasize greasy quantity over quality.
- Keep a regular schedule. Late-night dining* may be fashionable, but it's also most fattening. Unless you have a healthy snack earlier in the evening, you'll probably be too hungry by the time you order. When you are ravenous, you're more likely to order the wrong foods and overeat.
- Don't go hungry all day to save up for one big meal. You'll be starving come dinnertime. Instead, eat some high-quality protein and light snacks, such as salad or raw vegetables, throughout the day.
- Know exactly what you will order **before** you get to the restaurant. If necessary, review your Daily Food Diary or your PEP Blueprint before leaving home.
- Know the precise number of Bonus calories you have to spend, and what they will buy.
- Reserve your Bonus calories for extra foods or drinks you want to have, and spend only those Bonus calories that you have saved.
- Drink your complete water requirement for the evening **before** you eat. The cold water will reduce your appetite.
- Save your daily servings of fats and oils for dining out. While you must avoid fried foods, remember that most restaurant foods contain hidden fats and oils.
- To avoid temptation, order without looking at the menu. If you

*Food eaten after 10:00 P.M. may not metabolize properly and may end up as **fat**.

already know what you should eat, there's no need to confuse the issue at the last minute by poring over a tempting menu.

- Be assertive when ordering. Give clear, precise instructions about how you want your food prepared. Don't hesitate to send it back if it isn't right.
- If you like to have a cocktail, it's best to drink a glass of wine *with* dinner. Cocktails before dinner enhance your appetite, which could make you more likely to overeat.
- Don't eat a meal before a meal. In other words, steer clear of hors d'oeuvres. They are highly caloric and you can overeat before you know it. It's best to avoid them entirely. If you must, nibble on some fresh vegetable sticks—without the dip!
- Don't order a complete dinner. Soup, salad, bread, an entree with two vegetables, plus dessert, is just too much food. Instead, order a la carte. It's more sensible and you have greater control over what you get.
- Order a "doggie bag" at the *beginning* of the meal. Most restaurants serve portions that are too big. Ask the waiter to divide the food *before* you begin to eat, and place the extra portion into the "doggie bag." You won't be tempted to keep eating after you've had enough. Also, you may have tomorrow's lunch!
- If a "doggie bag" is unacceptable, perhaps you can split your entree with another person. If that is not possible, divide your food in half on the plate. Eat only one half and let the other half go to the garbage—better to waste than to waist.
- Avoid buffets. People usually eat too much at a buffet. If a buffet is unavoidable, take only one plate. Don't go through the line more than once. Choose plain fresh fruits, vegetables, and salads. Avoid dishes that are marinated, creamed, or dressed. Just because there are five different meats doesn't mean you should try them all. Take your normal portion of one item (or divide the portion between two things)—more than that will lead to a heaping plate. Don't put too much on your plate. Concentrate on leaving space between each different food on the plate.
- Eat the foods you like least first. They will take the edge off your hunger and are usually foods that are lower in calories.
- When you are invited to other people's homes to eat, don't feel afraid to tell them about your food requirements. Most hosts

and hostesses appreciate being told in advance. You might say, "I'm looking forward to your dinner party on Saturday. I want you to know that I don't eat sweets or salad dressings, so don't be offended if I don't polish everything off. You're such a great cook that a little of anything you make will be a real treat." If necessary, a simple, "No, thank you. I don't want any," will be the best defense against a food pusher.

Managing a Menu

When you are faced with ordering from a menu, here are some of the guidelines to help you make smart choices:

Appetizers

Order unsweetened fruit juice, consommé, broth, bouillon, a vegetable relish tray, or unsweetened fresh fruit cocktail.

Avoid deep-fried potatoes, appetizers with sweet sauces, puff pastries, creamed soups, sweetened fruit juices, and seafood cocktails (unless you plan to cut down the protein portion of your entree).

Soups

Order bouillon, broth, consommé, fish soups made without cream or *roux* (butter and flour for thickening), light vegetable soups, and most Oriental soups made without noodles or dumplings.

Avoid creamed soups and those that are thickened with *roux*. Have pea, bean, lentil, barley, noodle, or dumpling soups *only* when they are counted as your complex-carbohydrate allowance. And then, have only a small serving.

Salads

Order large vegetable salads and ask that dressing be served on the side so you can take a measured amount. Better, ask for vinegar or lemon instead of dressing. Fresh fruit salads and salads with plain seafood are good choices for a main meal.

Avoid salads that have been dressed, or those such as coleslaw, macaroni, egg, or tuna that are likely to be loaded with mayonnaise. Avoid fruit salads that have canned, sweetened fruit. Don't order Waldorf or other types of salad that use whipped cream. Avoid salads that offer sherbet. Pass up stuffed avocado halves, too.

Breads

Order any kind of bread as long as it is not sweetened, frosted, or glazed with sugar. Eat only the amount you are allowed. If you order toast, order it dry and ask for butter on the side. If you use butter, it must not exceed your fat allowance. Hard rolls, French bread, sourdough bread, rye, wheat, pumpernickel, and plain bagels are good choices.

Avoid biscuits, fried breads, fried tortillas, sweet breads, sweet rolls, and coffee cake.

Eggs

Order soft-boiled, poached, hard-boiled, or baked.

Avoid fried, scrambled, and eggs that have a sauce such as eggs Benedict (unless you specify that the sauce be omitted).

Vegetables

Order all the vegetables listed in Food Group 2. Have them steamed, if possible.

Avoid vegetables that are creamed, scalloped, au gratin, deep-fried, or stir-fried.

Potatoes

Order them steamed, boiled, mashed, or baked (using only the amount of butter or sour cream that you are allowed).

Avoid French fries, cottage fries, hash browns, au gratin, and scalloped potatoes.

Meat, Fish, and Chicken

Order roasted, broiled, boiled, baked, or charcoal-grilled.

Avoid fried, breaded, creamed, sauced, and scalloped. Trim away all fat. If you order bacon, order it flat and dry. Send it back if it's not right. Remember, bacon is a fat, not a meat.

Desserts

Order fresh fruits in season or fruit salads, without sugar or cream. You may have to order from the appetizer menu to get what you want.

Avoid desserts on the pastry cart. Don't order anything that contains sugar, fat, or flour. Don't order gelatins, puddings, custards, flan, or mousse.

Beverages

Order coffee, tea, nonfat milk, unsweetened fruit juices, mineral waters, diet sodas, plain water, iced tea, iced coffee; wine, liquor, light beer, or dry wine.

Avoid regular milk, coffees with cream or sugar added, liqueurs (after-dinner drinks), sweet wines, sugared soft drinks, sangria, lemonade, and sweetened fruit juices.

Slender Solutions:
Snowbird Travel Savvy

Well-traveled people know all the ins and outs that can make a rather ordinary trip really sensational.

It takes much the same kind of know-how to travel with style while maintaining your weight.

Most people are under the impression that travel automatically precludes weight maintenance.

The Snowbird Traveler explodes that myth.

Patients from the Southwest Bariatric Nutrition Center have proven time and again that travel can be both exciting *and* healthful. In fact, when the two go hand in hand, the pleasure of the trip is actually heightened.

You come home feeling enriched and renewed. There's a sense of accomplishment and self-satisfaction because you have remained in control.

Quite a difference from coming home with a depressing 10 extra pounds to deal with!

The first thing you should know is that you are not the first person to travel in a health-conscious style.

There are scores of finicky globe-trotters—some of them quite famous.

For example, did you know that Gloria Swanson never went anywhere without taking her own supply of bottled water?

Yul Brynner always traveled with his own mattress.

Toni Tennille, a strict vegetarian, frequents the world's best vegetarian restaurants when she's on the road.

Comedian-author Larry Wilde travels with his own salad bowl. In fact, one of his most memorable meals was an enormous California-style salad, a wedge of cheese, a freshly baked baguette, and a glass of wine. What made it so memorable? The salad was composed of spectacularly tasty French vegetables and was enhanced by a view of Paris from Larry's hotel balcony. It was a feast for all the senses!

A patient of mine from Minneapolis travels with a portable gym so that he can exercise in spite of an irregular schedule or inclement weather.

The point is, many people have devised seemingly unorthodox schemes for ensuring their own comfort and health while traveling.

There are many ways to travel in style without jeopardizing your figure or fitness.

Develop a style that will work for you.

The following guide for the Snowbird Traveler is designed to get you through some of the rough spots. It will spark some of your own ideas. You will soon discover that traveling and keeping fit are not mutually exclusive.

The Snowbird Traveler

Traveling by Air

- Request a special meal. Call the airline in advance and ask for a low-calorie or diabetic meal. It will probably be fresher and tastier than regular airline food. Be sure to remind the flight attendant of your special meal as you board the plane.
- If you can't abide airline food, take some sensible snacks in your carry-on bag: fruit, vegetable sticks, cold chicken, a light sandwich, et cetera.
- Skip airline peanuts, snacks, and cocktails unless you have saved enough Bonus calories to cover them. Most snacks are loaded with salt and sugar, so it's best to avoid them, period.
- If the flight is short, wait until you reach your destination, then have a more relaxed, enjoyable meal.

Traveling by Car

- Don't take fattening snacks in the car. Instead, carry an assortment of sugar-free mints and gum plus an assortment of low-calorie drinks: club soda, vegetable juices, coffee, tea, et cetera.
- Keep yourself busy with plenty to read, needlework, or correspondence (a portable lap desk is handy).
- Take exercise breaks. Stop periodically during the drive and do some stretching exercises or take a brisk walk.
- Avoid roadside fast-food spots. The food is usually short on nutrition and long on calories, loaded with fat, salt, and sugar.
- If you know there are no suitable restaurants along the way, take a light picnic.
- Carry your daily requirement of water in a thermos. Add a slice of lemon or lime and some ice cubes to keep it fresh-tasting.

Plan Ahead for Success

- Don't eat whenever the urge strikes. Make a master plan and stick to it. If there is likely to be street food you want to try, plan to have it *instead of a meal*. Decide how much you will eat *before* you get there. Then stick to your guns.

- Walk as much as possible. Take comfortable shoes for sightseeing, shopping, or taking in museums and galleries. Walking is the best way to get to know a city and keep in shape at the same time.
- Plan ahead to meet your exercise needs. The hotel where you stay may have workout facilities. If not, many hotels now offer maps with local, measured routes for walkers and joggers. If you travel very often, consider investing in a portable gym, which is a great help during bad weather. If all else fails, carry a jump rope in your suitcase.
- Take the proper clothing for exercising.
- If you are staying several days in one hotel, notify them ahead of time if you have specific food needs. Most establishments are happy to be of service.
- To find the kind of restaurants you need, inquire at the hotel, or consult local travel books or restaurant guides.
- It's a good idea to take an "emergency" or "convenience" kit. Include things you may need or want, such as packets of low-calorie dressing, decaffeinated tea, decaffeinated coffee, a portable coffee maker, a can/bottle opener, sugar-free mints and gum, and packets or cubes of bouillon. After you arrive you can buy a small supply of fresh vegetables or fruit for snacks, vegetable juice, bottled mineral water, fresh lemons or limes, et cetera. You might also consider having small cans of seafood or chicken for those times when you are either too tired or too busy to go to a restaurant.
- Plan to eat only one big or special meal per day. Don't have one restaurant's famous breakfast, another's special lunch, and another's gourmet dinner. Space them out, *one per day*. The rest of your meals should be light and nourishing—fruit, vegetables, salads with low-calorie dressing, and small portions of high-quality protein. Don't starve all day and overeat at night.
- Plan especially enjoyable activities for *after* meals. You won't be as tempted to overeat, and you can substitute the activity for dessert.

Slender Solutions:
Snowbird Tips for Enlightened Entertaining

It seems that entertaining should be the easiest situation of all to control, yet it often leads to real diet downfalls.

That's because so many people have the erroneous notion that stylish entertaining requires groaning boards of rich, elaborate, high-calorie foods.

Nothing could be further from the truth.

Today's entertaining doesn't have to follow the rigid dictates of yesteryear when more was thought to be better.

We are health-conscious today.

Less is more.

We regard quality more highly than quantity.

Simplicity is the key. Fine food simply prepared is the most creative offering you can give.

It shows respect for yourself and for your guests.

Keep in mind that preparing the same good food for your guests as you do for yourself also shows care and consideration. You'll be surprised how many guests will appreciate your approach. It may encourage them to do the same.

They will be able to enjoy the company and conversation. Better, they won't secretly curse you for days afterward as they struggle to lose the extra weight they gained at your party.

Presenting food that is delicious, creatively prepared, and health-conscious is perhaps the most loving gesture you can make toward your friends and family.

As you learned from the Snowbird Diet, fine food does not have to be boring. In fact, it can easily be exotic and exciting.

Even at that, it's time you start deemphasizing food. After all, you are not inviting friends over because you want to concentrate on food. You are looking for stimulating conversation and a lively interchange between people. Food is just one small part of the evening.

Here are Snowbird's tips for today's more enlightened entertaining:

- Serve foods that fit your Personal Eating Plan. The selection is practically limitless. Don't make something you can't enjoy, too.

Nobody feels comfortable when the host or hostess doesn't eat.

- Plan a very short predinner cocktail period. Serve light drinks and calorie-conscious appetizers. A magnificent basket of fresh *crudités* with a low-calorie dip is not only ideal, it is beautiful. Be sure to have plenty of nonalcoholic and sugar-free drinks on hand.
- Adapt your favorite recipes to make them lower in calories and fat (see the guidelines later in this chapter). For other ideas, browse through any of the many new cookbooks devoted to light cooking.
- While you are preparing the food, sip a glass of carbonated water with lime to keep yourself from nibbling (it also keeps your palate cleansed for tasting). If you really have to nibble, keep an assortment of sliced raw vegetables in a plastic bag in the refrigerator. Having them prepared in advance is a great help in deterring more damaging nibbles.
- Be sure to allow plenty of time for all the preparation, and get as much help as you can for serving and cleanup. Stress and fatigue can trigger overeating. Plan a menu that will allow you to enjoy the party.
- Instead of serving something sinful for dessert, base your selection on fresh fruit. Poached pears, fresh berries in season with a splash of liqueur, or a layered fresh fruit salad are elegant and delicious. For those who would like to be more indulgent, you might offer small cookies or pastries that have been purchased in a small amount just for the occasion. If you don't bake them, you won't be as tempted to nibble.
- As for the leftovers, send home "doggie bags" with your guests. Otherwise, freeze leftovers immediately for later use. **Don't** tempt yourself by keeping them in the refrigerator.

Shopping Smart

How many times have you eaten something so that it wouldn't go to waste? Instead of ending up in the garbage, it ended up on you.

Developing smart shopping strategy can help you avoid overbuying, which often leads to overeating.

Here are some hints to help you shop for slimness:

- Make a detailed shopping list based on foods from your Personal Eating Plan. Buy only what is on the list. Don't buy foods you shouldn't eat "just in case" or "just for the family." Let everyone benefit from your good nutrition habits.
- Don't shop too often. Try to consolidate trips by planning ahead and making a complete list—every three to seven days should be enough. Pick a time of day to shop when you are not hungry or tired and can go without your spouse or children.
- Shop the perimeter of the market. That's where the fresh meat, vegetables, fruit, and dairy products are located. Steer clear of the center aisles that are loaded with snack foods and sweets. If there is something you must have, park your cart and walk down the aisle to pick it up. Don't cruise the aisle tossing junk food into your basket.
- Buy absolutely the best-quality food your budget will allow. If you cut down the quantity, you can afford better quality. The only exceptions to this are prime meats that should be avoided because of their high fat content.
- Buy an abundance of fresh vegetables. Wash them and have them ready for emergency snacks or to extend a meal when you are extra hungry. Have frozen vegetables on hand for emergencies.

Adapting Recipes Snowbird-Style

Low-calorie cooking is the most refined of all cooking styles.

Because it relies on the true taste of fresh, fine ingredients, it requires care and good judgment in its preparation.

None of the flavors are disguised with fats, sugars, breaded coatings, or rich sauces.

Poor-quality food cannot be dressed up to taste as though it is decent without the benefit of fattening tricks.

So for low-calorie food to be delicious, you have to start with the best.

Here are some of the ways you can trim the fat from some of your favorite recipes without changing the flavor, *if* you start with the freshest and best available ingredients:

- Look for ways to decrease the fat content of the recipe. Since fat is the most concentrated form of calories, cutting down a little will make a big difference.
- Steam vegetables rather than sauté, and serve them with wedges of lemon instead of butter or oil.
- Sauté foods using a trace amount of butter or oil, making up the difference by using a nonstick pan and adding a bit of light stock, sherry, or dry wine to the pan.
- Use nonfat milk products exclusively.
- Substitute plain, low-fat yoghurt for sour cream whenever possible.
- Use half the amount of mayonnaise a recipe calls for, making up the difference with plain, low-fat yoghurt.
- Brown food without fat by using a heavy skillet with a nonstick coating. Drain fatty foods on paper towels to degrease them.
- Remove all visible fat from meats and poultry before cooking.
- Never fry foods.
- Cook meats on a rack so that excess fats can drain away.
- Pop corn in a microwave or a hot-air popper rather than in oil.
- Refrigerate broths, stocks, and soups before serving so that the congealed fat can rise to the top and easily be removed.
- Season foods with fresh herbs, spices, and lemon instead of adding butter or oil.
- Serve more fish, seafood, and poultry (without skin), and less pork and red meat. When choosing meats, always buy the leanest cuts. Avoid prime meats.
- Use a gravy strain or a soup strain to pour off excess fat from pan juices, stock, et cetera.

Look for ways to cut the sugar content of recipes. The total amount of sugar can usually be cut by 1/3 or 1/2 without really affecting the flavor.

- For desserts, use fresh fruits or those that are canned or frozen without sugar added.
- Replace all or part of the sugar in a recipe with a sugar substitute. This may not be entirely successful with some baked goods, but it works beautifully with most other types of sweets, including puddings, custards, gelatins, and so on.

- Use natural, unsweetened fruit juice (such as apple or pine-apple) as a sweetener instead of sugar.
- Unsweetened fruit butters are a lovely substitute for jams, jellies, or syrup.

Other Calorie-Cutting Tips

- Be accurate about portion size. No recipe is low-calorie if you eat a double portion.
- Plan meals that include low-calorie fillers such as soups, big salads, and nonstarchy vegetables.
- Use puréed, low-calorie fillers rather than flour as a thickening agent.
- Unless you are certain of their caloric content, avoid prepackaged foods.
- For sauces, reduce strained pan juices with a little lemon juice, dry sherry, or dry wine. Herbs, minced garlic, or minced shallots will add pizzazz.
- Herbs, spices, and natural extracts add lots of flavor to cooking without adding calories.
- Most calories in wine or sherry evaporate with the alcohol when they are cooked.
- Slice bread thinly or buy it thinly sliced. Remove the doughy centers from hard rolls and eat mostly crust.
- Accent food with a variety of low-calorie condiments, such as mustards, pickles, steak sauces, capers, green peppercorns, et cetera.

12

Snowbird Dieters
Ask the Doctor

Q: *Usually I get very depressed when I go on a diet. How can I avoid this?*

A: Studies have shown that depression can be directly related to blood sugar or deprivation of food intake and variety. Since the Snowbird Diet carefully regulates blood sugar by lowering insulin, you should not be bothered by erratic mood swings. Also, the food prescribed in this diet is so uncommonly tasty and interesting that you won't feel deprived—a common complaint of dieters.

Q: *Should I go on the Snowbird Diet while I'm pregnant?*

A: This is one of the most important times in your life. While the diet is nutritionally sound, your special requirements may not be met on this program. You should abide by the advice of your obstetrician and his nutritionist. They are aware of any special problems you may have.

Q: *Is it advisable for my teenage daughter to go on the Snowbird Diet?*

A: Because the rates at which teens grow and mature are so vastly different, I recommend you consult your physician before placing your child on *any* special diet. However, since the Snowbird Diet is so well balanced, it is generally fine for most teens.

275

Q: *What should I do if I'm still hungry after a meal?*

A: Assuming you ate absolutely everything prescribed for that meal, you simply should not be *hungry.* If you want food, it means your appetite is running amok!

Remember, once food is eaten, it takes twenty minutes before the brain gives the signal that you feel full.

Wait twenty minutes before eating anything else.

Leave the table immediately so that you aren't tempted to pick at leftovers. Remove yourself from the sight and smell of all food.

Brush your teeth and rinse with an astringent mouthwash.

Take a few deep breaths, walk around the block, or do some simple stretches.

Drink a glass of water. If you still feel the urge to put something in your mouth, have a cold carbonated beverage (no sugar or caffeine). Sip it slowly through a straw.

Remember: This kind of hunger is purely psychological. Your *appetite* is needy, but in reality you are not *hungry.* Do anything that will take your mind off food. Be assured that the feeling is only temporary. It will pass quickly, and you'll be happy you didn't succumb to that old urge to stuff yourself. While an "appetite attack" is normal for most dieters (especially at first), these simple techniques will help the appetite fade for good.

Q: *Is it true that when you have food cravings, something is missing in your diet?*

A: No. In fact, most food cravings are either cultural or psychological and don't correlate in any way with nutritional needs.

Q: *What if I'm really hungry for something forbidden?*

A: If you're on maintenance, you can save up for it (see Bonus PEP in chapter 10). However, if you haven't yet reached your goal, don't permit your brain to indulge in food fantasies—thoughts are fattening.

Instead, change activities. Avoid those that involve food—reading recipes or magazines with lots of food ads. If you're watching TV and tempting food commercials come on, simply get up and leave the room. Remember, *head hunger* is your **enemy.** Your system must learn to respond only when you *need* food, not whenever you *want* it.

Q: *What if I absolutely don't like something that's on the 12-day menu plan?*

A: Refer to the Emergency Food Plan and simply swap a *like meal* for a *like meal.* For instance, if you don't want Tuesday's dinner, you can exchange it for the Tuesday dinner on the Emergency Food Plan. **Don't** swap a Friday lunch for a Wednesday dinner, or a Monday dinner for a Thursday dinner, et cetera. You must trade a like for a like—a Saturday lunch for a Saturday lunch and so on.

Q: *Why is it so important to exchange a like meal for a like meal? Why can't I substitute a Tuesday lunch for a Friday lunch?*

A: The meals are delicately balanced and paced throughout the entire 12-day plan, providing specific nutrients exactly in the sequence in which they should be for maximum energy and weight loss. If you start swapping meals willy-nilly, the entire program may be in jeopardy. Save your creative menu planning for maintenance, where nutritional balance won't be quite as critical.

Q: *Does food prepared in advance lose all its nutrients?*

A: Not necessarily. If you cook food in a manner that will retain its vitamins (steaming, cooking *en papillote*, et cetera), then store it well covered, it should retain most of its vitamins (minerals are never lost).

For maximum nutrition, buy the freshest food available. Food can lose much of its nutritional value as it lingers on the store shelf.

Q: *What if my religion prevents me from eating something prescribed on the menu plan?*

A: Refer to the Emergency Food Plan and substitute the meal you can't eat for the corresponding meal for the corresponding day.

Q: *I have a problem with constipation. What should I do?*

A: Drinking an adequate amount of water should relieve constipation. This, along with regular exercise and a balanced diet, may clear up the problem entirely. However, if you still need help, take 2 tablespoons of unrefined bran (not bran cereal) mixed with hot water to a consistency that is palatable.

Take this in the morning before breakfast along with your water regimen.

Q: *Will massive weight loss make me look older or haggard?*

A: If you do everything exactly as prescribed—drink water, eat *all* your food, and exercise daily—your skin should be resilient, your body tone will improve, and you will actually look years younger. However, this obviously depends to a certain extent on your age and general physical condition.

Q: *Diets make me feel so tired. Is the Snowbird Diet any different?*

A: Many contemporary diets are based on faulty information and lack the proper nutritional balance for maximum weight loss and maximum energy—both of which are critical to the dieter. If you practice the Snowbird Diet exactly as prescribed, you will feel better than you have in years, with energy to spare because your body will be in correct nutritional balance.

Q: *What can I do to get rid of cellulite?*

A: The Snowbird Diet is an ideal solution for people who are troubled with cellulite, because it combines two essentials—balanced diet and exercise. Women are more likely to have cellulite than are men, due to different hormone levels and even heredity. Cellulite is nothing more than layers of fatty tissues, one on top of the other. Once fat builds up, circulation gets sluggish. Aerobic exercise is a wonderful solution because it burns lots of calories and improves circulation at the same time.

People who are sedentary are also more likely to get cellulite. If you sit a lot, it's important to move around at least once an hour. This will increase circulation. Also, avoid wearing tight clothing that might restrict blood flow. Vigorous professional massage is also beneficial.

One easy and often successful method to get rid of cellulite is to walk up stairs two or more at a time. This stretches the back of the thigh, where cellulite most commonly occurs in women, and no other type of exercise seems to provide the necessary stretching and muscle tension at that spot. However, don't try to do this all at once. Start one step at a time up one flight. Then two at a time up one flight. Then two at a time up two flights, and so on. The more this is done the quicker the cellulite will disappear in most people. I have seen a modest amount of cellulite completely disappear in a female patient using this technique of walking up three flights of stairs, two at a time, every day during a two-week vacation. But again, be careful to do this gradually because any amount of unaccustomed activity should be gradually increased until the results are accomplished.

Q: *You list tomatoes as a vegetable. I always thought a tomato was a fruit.*

A: You are correct. The tomato is a fruit. However, most people use it like a vegetable, and its caloric content is similar to that of the vegetables on the Group 2 list, making it interchangeable with vegetables.

Q: *I'm 50 pounds overweight and I'm desperate. What about using one of the protein powders advertised in some health food stores and the newspapers?*

A: Although there are many products that promise spectacular results, there is only one I would feel safe in recommending. The product is Optifast made by Sandoz Nutrition Corporation. It is part of a total program used and researched at Cleveland's Mt. Sinai Medical Center by Victor Vertes, M.D. and staff. Optifast is the name of the protein supplement used in this program which is successful, safe, and fully researched. The program is only available through certified physicians and has data on over one million patient/weeks experience to prove its success and safety. A doctor can show you how to combine Optifast with the Snowbird Diet. Do not use it without a doctor's supervision.

Q: *What should I do if I have not lost all the desired weight at the end of the twelfth day?*

A: As this is a nutritionally sound diet, continue taking the appropriate vitamin and calcium supplements and simply return to the first day of the diet. Repeat as often as necessary.

If you are interested in a newsletter dealing with body-weight control, luxury health-oriented vacations, and fitness and health, write to:

> Southwest Bariatric Nutrition Center
> 6925 5th Avenue, Suite E
> Scottsdale, Arizona 85251

BIBLIOGRAPHY

EXERCISE

Anderson, B. *Stretching.* Bolinas, Calif.: Shelter Publications, 1980.

Bailey, C. *Fit or Fat.* Boston: Houghton Mifflin, 1978.

Cooper, K. H. *The Aerobics Program for Total Well-Being.* New York: M. Evans, 1982.

McArdle, W. D., F. Katch, and V. Katch. *Exercise Physiology, Energy, Nutrition, and Human Performance.* Philadelphia, PA.: Lea and Febiger, 1981.

Wilmore, J. H. *The Wilmore Fitness Program, a Personalized Guide to Total Fitness and Health.* New York: Simon & Schuster, 1981.

Vodak, P. *Exercise, the Why and the How.* Palo Alto, Calif.: Bull Publishing, 1980.

Wood, P. *California Diet and Exercise Program.* Mountain View, Calif.: World Books, 1983.

PSYCHOLOGICAL AWARENESS

Burns, D. D. *Feeling Good.* New York: William Morrow, 1980.

Cordell, F. D., and G. R. Giebler. *Psychological War on Fat.* Niles, Ill.: Argus, 1977.

Harris, T. A. *I'm OK—You're OK*. New York: Harper and Row, 1969.

Lazarus, A. A. *Multimodal Behavior Therapy: BASIC ID*. New York: Springer, 1976.

Peters, T. J., and R. H. Waterman, Jr. *In Search of Excellence*. New York: Harper and Row, 1982.

Smith, M. J. *When I Say No, I Feel Guilty*. New York: Bantam Books, 1975.

MAINTENANCE

Kraus, B. *Calories and Carbohydrates*, 5th edition. New York: New American Library, 1983.

Editors of *Consumer Guide*. *The Dieter's Complete Guide to . . . Calories, Carbohydrates, Sodium, Fats and Cholesterol*. Skokie, Ill.: Publications International, 1981.

Pennington, J. A. T., and H. N. Church. *Food Values of Portions Commonly Used*, 13th edition. New York: Harper and Row, 1980.

LeGette, Bernard. *LeGette's Calorie Encyclopedia*. New York: Warner Books, 1983.

U.S.D.A. *Handbook of the Nutritional Contents of Foods*. New York: Dover Publications, 1975.

National Research Council, Committee on Dietary Allowances, Food and Nutrition Board. *Recommended Dietary Allowances*, 9th edition. Washington, D.C.: National Academy of Sciences, 1980.

American Diabetes Association, American Dietetic Association. *Exchange Lists for Meal Planning*, 1976.

GENERAL HEALTH AND NUTRITION

Barrett, S. *The Health Robbers*. 2nd edition. Philadelphia: George F. Stickley, 1980.

Johnson, G. T. *The Harvard Medical School Health Letter*. Boston: Harvard Medical School.

White, A., and Society for Nutrition Education. *The Family Health Cookbook*. New York: David McKay, 1980.

Deutsch, R. M. *The Family Guide to Better Food and Better Health.* New York: Bantam Books, 1982.

McGill, M., and O. Pye. *The No-Nonsense Guide to Food and Nutrition.* Piscataway, NJ: New Century Pub., 1982.

Cumming, C., and V. Newman. *Eater's Guide, Nutrition Basics for Busy People.* Englewood Cliffs, NJ: Prentice-Hall, 1981.

For a more extensive list of books on the subject, write to
Nutrition References and Book Reviews
Chicago Nutrition Association
8158 South Kedzie Ave.
Chicago, IL 60652

REFERENCES

Burns, D. D. *Feeling Good.* New York: William Morrow, 1980.

Cordell, F. D., and G. R. Giebler. *Psychological War on Fat.* Niles, Ill.: Argus, 1977.

Harris, T. A. *I'm OK—You're OK.* New York: Harper and Row, 1969.

Lazarus, A. A. *Multimodal Behavior Therapy: BASIC ID.* New York: Springer, 1976.

Peters, T. J., and R. H. Waterman, Jr. *In Search of Excellence.* New York: Harper and Row, 1982.

Smith, M. J. *When I Say No, I Feel Guilty.* New York: Bantam Books, 1975.

Index

Calories:
  Bonus PEP, 222–23, 236, 240, 245, 246, 262, 268, 276
  consumed on the Snowbird Diet, 48, 61
  counting, 14, 220, 221
  in individual recipes, *see individual recipes*
  intake and expenditure, 15–16, 162, 241
  for Substitute Emergency Meal, 158
Canadian bacon, 86, 126
Cancer, 166, 168
Cannellini beans, turkey scallopini with, 109
Carbohydrates, 14, 48
  complex, food group, 225, 248, 251–52
  in individual recipes, *see individual recipes*
  refined (simple), 41, 49, 52
  for Substitute Emergency Meal, 148
  Cardiorespiratory exercise *see* Aerobic exercise
  Cardiovascular system, 19, 21, 22–26, 41, 52*n*.
  diseases of, and Snowbird Diet program, 166–68
  stress-related illness, 197
  stress test, 168, 171
Carotid pulse, 176–77
Carrot(s):
  choucroute, 141–42
  scallops and sole in white wine, 129
  toss, 117
Car travel, 268
Caviar, 108
  consommé, 73
  omelette, 108
Cellulite, 278–79
Cereals, 251
Champagne, raspberries in, 100
Cheese, *see* Dairy food group; Milk; Protein, food group; *individual cheeses*
Chèvre:
  smoked salmon omelette, 88
  and spinach omelette, 100–101
  Stobo castle salad, 114–15
  and tomato on flatbread, 78
Chicken, 266
  and artichoke hearts with mushrooms, 136
  broth, *see* Broth, chicken
  ginger, 67–68
  pita, 229
  Snowbird salad, 140–41
Chinese pea pods, steamed fresh, 68
Cholesterol levels, blood, 22, 24, 167, 168
Choucroute, 141–42
Cilantro leaves for emerald soup, 127
Clothing, 278
  exercise, 30, 185, 193–94, 195, 269
Coffee, 45, 60–61, 62, 266
Colitis, 197
Commitment, 31
Comparing yourself to others, 208
Complex carbohydrates food group, 225, 248, 251–52
Concentration problems, 197, 202

Condiments, 274
Consommé:
  caviar, 73
  hot Virgin Bloody Bull, 86–87
Constipation, 11, 39, 168, 277
Convenience of a diet, 9, 11
"Convenience" kit for travel, 269
Cooking methods, 60, 253, 277
  adapting recipes, 272–74
Cooking of Southwest France (Wolfert), 13
Cool-down exercises, 189–90
Cornish game hen(s):
  cold, 94
  Dijonnaise, 89
Crackers, 252
  see also Lahvosh
Cranberry(ies):
  blend, 134
  creamy baked apples, 117
Cranberry Cocktail, Low-Cal, 61
Cranberry Spritzer, Low-Cal, 61
Cravings, 276
  see also Appetite; Hunger
Cucumber:
  curried yoghurt soup, hot, 94
  Sonora salad, 122
Curry powder, 56
  curried yoghurt soup, hot, 94–95
Cutting back on Snowbird menus, 62

Dairy food group, 225, 246–47
Day 1 to Day 12 of the Snowbird Diet, menus and recipes for, 65–143
Decaffeinated drinks, 45
Depression, 10, 165, 169, 196, 275
  the urge to eat and, 199, 200, 204
Desserts, 266, 269
Diary, *see* Food diary
Diet soft drinks, 45–46, 61, 266
Dining out, 144–45, 220, 260–66, 269
  managing a menu, 264–66
  mental imagery to prepare for, 260–61
  tips for, 261–64
Dinner, *see* Menus and recipes
Distribution plans, food, 228–36, 245
Diuretics, 38
Dizziness, 42
"Doggie bag," 263, 271
Dressings, 145
  see also individual salads
Drugs, *see* Medications

Eating habits, 16–17, 26, 52–54
  binge eating, *see* Binge eating
  goof-proofing your surroundings, 28–30
Eating less and enjoying it more, 52–53
Eggs, 66, 140, 265
  omelette(s):
    caviar, 108
    chèvre and spinach, 100–101
    smoked salmon, 88